MIAMI WINTER SYMPOSIA — VOLUME 6

The Role of Cyclic Nucleotides in Carcinogenesis

edited by
J. Schultz
H. G. Gratzner

THE PAPANICOLAOU CANCER RESEARCH INSTITUTE

MIAMI, FLORIDA

*Proceedings of the Miami Winter Symposia, January 18-19, 1973,
organized by The Papanicolaou Cancer Research Institute, Miami, Florida*

ACADEMIC PRESS   New York and London 1973

A Subsidiary of Harcourt Brace Jovanovich, Publishers

ACADEMIC PRESS, INC.
111 Fifth Avenue, New York, New York 10003

United Kingdom Edition published by
ACADEMIC PRESS, INC. (LONDON) LTD.
24/28 Oval Road, London NW1

Library of Congress Cataloging in Publication Data
Main entry under title:

The Role of cyclic nucleotides in carcinogenesis.

(Miami winter symposia, v.   6)
"Proceedings of the Miami winter symposia, January
18-19, 1973, organized by the Papanicolaou Cancer
Research Institute, Miami."
        1.   Carcinogenesis–Congresses.   2.   Cyclic adenylic
acid–Congresses.   3.   Adenyl cyclase–Congresses.
I.   Schultz, Julius, DATE   ed.   II.   Gratzner, H. G.,
ed.   III.   Papanicolaou Cancer Research Institute.
IV.   Series. [DNLM: 1.   Carcinogens–Congresses.
2.   Nucleotides–Congresses.   W3 MI202 v. 6   1973.
XNLM: [QZ 202 R745 1973]]
RC268.5.R64 1973   616.9'94'071   72-9939
ISBN 0–12–632750–5

CONTENTS

CONTENTS

SPEAKERS, CHAIRMEN, AND DISCUSSANTS

C. Abell, University of Texas, Galveston, Texas

S. Assaf, University of Miami School of Medicine, Miami, Florida

H. Baer, University of Alberta, Edmonton, Canada

A. Berg, Medical College of Pennsylvania, Philadelphia, Pennsylvania

M. W. Bitensky, Yale University, New Haven, Connecticut

M. Blecher, Georgetown University, Washington, D. C.

P. Bornstein, University of Washington, Seattle, Washington

Z. Brada, Papanicolaou Cancer Research Institute, Miami, Florida

P. Brown, Brown University, Providence, Rhode Island

M. Chasin, The Squibb Institute for Medical Research, Princeton, New Jersey

G. Cherayil, Medical College of Wisconsin, Milwaukee, Wisconsin

W. Y. Cheung, St. Jude's Children's Research Hospital, Memphis, Tennessee

C. Dalton, Hoffman-La Roche, Inc., Nutley, New Jersey

J. Fessenden-Raden, Cornell University, Ithaca, New York

P. A. Galand, Free University of Brussels, Brussels, Belgium

G. N. Gill, University of California, San Diego, California

R. A. Hickie, University of Saskatchewan, Canada

S. L. Hsia, University of Miami School of Medicine, Miami, Florida

A. Hsie, Oak Ridge National Laboratory, Oak Ridge, Tennessee

G. S. Johnson, National Institutes of Health, Bethesda, Maryland

R. A. Johnson, Vanderbilt University, Nashville, Tennessee

M. Klein, New York University, New York, New York

J. Kowal, University Hospitals, Cleveland, Ohio

G. Krishna, National Institutes of Health, Bethesda, Maryland

R.C. Leif, Papanicolaou Cancer Research Institute, Miami, Florida

R. W. Longton, NMRI, NNMC, Bethesda, Maryland

M. Lubin, Dartmouth Medical School, Hanover, New Hampshire

K. S. McCarty, Duke Medical Center, Durham, North Carolina

L. Mandel, Merck Institute, Rahway, New Jersey

J. Miller, ICN Nucleic Acid Research Institute, Irvine, California

C. Moore, UTMB and AECOM, Bronx, New York

J. Neumann, Boston University, Boston, Massachusetts

I. Pastan (Session Chairman), National Institutes of Health, Bethesda, Maryland

K. N. Prasad, University of Colorado, Denver, Colorado

T. T. Puck (Session Chairman), University of Colorado, Denver, Colorado

A. Réthy, University of Debrecen, Debrecen, Hungary

D. R. Robinson, Massachusetts General Hospital, Boston, Massachusetts

J. Roth, University of Connecticut, Storrs, Connecticut

W. L. Ryan, University of Nebraska, Lincoln, Nebraska

J. Schultz, Papanicolaou Cancer Research Institute, Miami, Florida

W. Sheifert, Salk Institute, San Diego, California

R. Sharma, Veterans Administration Hospital, Memphis, Tennessee

H. Sheppard, Hoffman-La Roche, Inc., Nutley, New Jersey

J. R. Sheppard, University of Colorado, Denver, Colorado

E. E. Smith, Boston University School of Medicine, Boston, Massachusetts

S. Strada, University of Texas, Houston, Texas

H. Tai, New York University, New York, New York

C. Tihon, St. Louis University, St. Louis, Missouri

V. Tomasi, University of Ferrara, Ferrara, Italy

J. J. Voorhees (Session Chairman), University of Michigan, Ann Arbor, Michigan

G. Weber (Session Chairman), Indiana University, Indianapolis, Indiana

W. D. Wicks, University of Colorado, Denver, Colorado

A. Wollenberger, Academy of Science of the G.D.R., Berlin, Germany

C. Zeilig, Vanderbilt University, Nashville, Tennessee

PREFACE

When the directors of the Symposia first organized the program in 1969, they named it "The Biochemistry-PCRI Symposia", inasmuch as Dr. Whelan was Chairman of the Department of Biochemistry of the University of Miami and Dr. Schultz was Director of the Papanicolaou Cancer Research Institute. However, as time has gone on and the popularity of the Symposia increased, it became rather difficult to refer to the Biochemistry-PCRI Symposia since it had no local identification. We therefore began calling it informally the Miami Winter Symposia, by which title it will be known from this year on.

Previous volumes will be considered as starting in 1970. Volume 1 in 1970 and Volume 2 in 1971 included both symposia. In 1972 each symposium was published as a separate volume (Volumes 3 and 4). This year the program organized by Biochemistry will be Volume 5 and this publication will be Volume 6. Those papers presented at the 1969 Symposia that were related to the phagocytic process, selected by J. Schultz, were published as a paperback titled "Biochemistry of the Phagocytic Process." This therefore bears no volume number.

The present volume constitutes the first symposium concerned with cyclic nucleotides and cancer. In a few short years the number of biological phenomena in which cyclic AMP has been implicated is indeed astounding. So it is not surprising that workers involved in the study of neoplasia have become immersed in experimentation involving the cyclic nucleotides, cyclases, and phosphodiesterases and their relationship to control of cellular proliferation and differentiation.

The observations which are reported in this volume can be termed the "biological" effects of cyclic nucleotides. The companion symposium, published as Volume 5 of this series, deals with protein phosphorylation, particularly as mediated by cyclic AMP. It is hoped that it will be possible in the not too distant future to identify each of the striking biological effects on cells induced by alteration in cyclic nucleotide levels with a specific molecular interaction, at a particular stage of the cell cycle, as exemplified by the topics covered in Volume 5. Such knowledge will be essential for an elucidation of the aberrations of cellular control manifested as cancer and other human proliferative diseases.

ACKNOWLEDGMENTS

We wish to acknowledge the financial support contributed by Eli Lily, Squibb and Company, Smith, Kline and French, and the NIH General Research Support Grant No. S01–RR 05690–02.

Finally, the suggestions made by Drs. J. Pastan and G. Weber are greatly appreciated. Special recognition is due the girls in the "boiler room" who transcribed the discussions and worked so hard to follow up the edited comments to be included in time for the publication.

J. Schultz
H. G. Gratzner

The Role of Cyclic Nucleotides in Carcinogenesis

CHEMICAL CARCINOGENESIS AND CYCLIC AMP

Wayne L. Ryan and Gary L. Curtis
University of Nebraska College of Medicine
Omaha, Nebraska   68105

The apparent rigorous control which is exercised over cell division in each organ led to the assumption that there exist substances in tissues which regulate cell division. This hypothesis usually has suggested that such compounds should act as inhibitors and that cells will divide at a maximal rate in the absence of the inhibitor. A search for such substances led us to investigate adenosine 3',5'-monophosphate (cyclic AMP) as a potential regulator of cell division.

Cyclic AMP was found to inhibit cell division in tissue culture and to do so in a unique manner. There is no apparent toxicity, such as detachment from the glass, even at concentrations of up to 3 mM. Removal of the cyclic AMP-containing medium permits the cells to divide again in a normal manner (1). The variety of means available for elevating the levels of cyclic AMP by means of adenylate cyclase and lowering the levels by phosphodiesterase permit cyclic AMP the requited flexibility to carry out this possible role as a regulator of cell division.

Considerable evidence has accumulated which suggests a correlation between the cellular level of cyclic AMP and the rate of cell division (2-5). A further development has been the comparison of the levels of cyclic AMP, or one or more of the enzymes of the cyclic AMP system in normal, transformed, or malignant cells (6-14). At present, most evidence indicates that the rapidly dividing cell has lower levels of cyclic AMP, and for this reason it is concluded that the transformed and malignant cell may have defects in the cyclic AMP system.

1

Although transformation of cells in vitro results in a number of interesting cellular changes, none of these changes seem to be uniquely associated with tumorigenicity or neoplasia (15, 16). For this reason, cell lines of known tumorigenicity and lineage were sought. An appropriate cell system for studying the changes in the cyclic AMP system following chemical carcinogenesis is that of Freeman et al (17). A normal rat embryo cell line, Flll, free of murine viruses, was transformed in vitro by a variety of chemical carcinogens and by the Rauscher Leukemia Virus. The resultant cell lines produce tumors in the neonatal rat. In addition, the normal rat embryo cell of origin is available for comparison with the tumorigenic cell lines (Figure 1).

The aim of this study is to assay the cyclic AMP system in normal and carcinogenic treated cells. In addition, investigations of the response of the tumor cell in vitro to cyclic AMP and cyclic AMP elevating agents may provide a rational basis for an approach to inhibiting the growth of the tumors produced in vivo by these cell lines.

MATERIALS AND METHODS
Cell Culture

The rat embryo cell lines (Flll p. 32-34, F1706 p. 118-122, F1849 p. 59-62, and F2412 p. 36-37) were seeded in 20 X 100 mm plastic culture dishes (Falcon) at a cell density of 5000/cm^2 in Dulbecco's Modified Eagle's Medium with glutamine (Grand Island Biological) with 10% fetal calf serum. To the medium was also added sodium bicarbonate (13.5 g/1), amphotercin B (2 mg/1), penicillin (50,000 units/1), and streptomycin (500 mg/1). The cells were incubated at 37° in an atmosphere of 5% CO_2 and 95% air. The cells were removed from the dishes with 0.25% trypsin. All cells were counted on a Model Fn Coulter Counter.

The inhibition studies were conducted in 60 mm petri dishes containing 5 ml. of Dulbecco's Modified Eagle's Medium with 10% fetal calf serum. The percent inhibition=

$$\frac{\text{Cell count (control)} - \text{cell count (treated)}}{\text{Cell count (control)}} \times 100$$

Adenylate Cyclase

After removing the culture medium, the cells were washed with 10 ml. of 0.85% saline. For values obtained at 24 hours, 48 hours, and 96 hours of incubation, the cells were removed by scraping. For the zero time value the cells were removed by trypsinization and 3 ml. of fetal calf serum added to inhibit the action of trypsin. After removal, the cells were centrifuged and the cells were prepared as described by Makman with the exception that 5 mM dithioerythritol was added to the buffer (13, 17).

The incubation conditions were modified from those described by Makman and Krishna and were determined to give linear rates of activity for 20 min. at 30° C (13, 17, 18). Incubations were carried out in 10 X 75 mm test tubes containing: 1.0 mM ^{3}H ATP, 4.5 mM $MgCl_2$, 2.0 mM cyclic AMP, 2.5 mM phosphoenolpyruvate, 3.0 mM theophylline, 1.25 mg/ml pyruvate kinase, 45 mM Tris-HCl pH 7.6, and either 8 mM NaF or the Tris-Mg buffers in a final volume of 200 µl. The reactions were started by addition of cell homogenates to give final concentrations ranging from 1.0 to 2.0 mg. protein per milliliter of assay. Incubations were carried out at 30° C and were terminated by the addition of 0.2 milliliter of 50 mM Tris/HCl, pH 7.6, 5 mM cyclic AMP, and 3 mM ATP. The reaction mixtures were heated for two minutes in a boiling water bath after which 0.6 ml. of distilled water was added per tube. The cyclic AMP was isolated and measured as described by Krishna (18).

Cyclic AMP Assay

The medium was removed from the cells and drained as completely as possible. To each dish of cells was added 5 ml. of 0.5 N perchloric acid in 25% ethanol (v/v) containing tracer cyclic AMP for estimation of recovery. The precipitated cell sheet was scraped, washed, and centrifuged. The supernatant was neutralized with saturated KOH. After removal of the precipitate, the supernatant was chromatographed by the method of Brooker (19). The cyclic AMP assay was used as described by Gilman (20). A sample from each series was treated with phosphodiesterase

3.

as described by Otten et al (4).

Cell Volume Determinations

For cell volume determinations, the growth media was removed from exponentially growing monolayer cultures and replaced with fresh growth media containing the test reagents. Following incubation, the cells were washed with 2 ml. Dulbecco's Tris buffer (0.025 M Tris, 0.1 M KH_2PO_4, and 0.25 M saline, pH 6.8-7.0) then incubated with 1 ml. of 0.25% trypsin for 5 minutes at 37°. The detached cells from each plate were placed in 100 ml. of Dulbecco's Modified Eagle's Medium, pH 7.2, (containing 0.04 M Tris buffer) supplemented with 10% fetal calf serum, penicillin (500 units/ml.), and streptomycin (500 g/ml.) and the cell volume measured with a Model B Coulter Counter.

RESULTS

In Figure 1 is a summary of some of the characteristics of four of the rat embryo cell lines. The most rapidly dividing cell is the F2412, which was transformed by 3-methylcholanthrene. The cell volume of the two transformed cell lines (F2412 and F1849) is very similar, and the largest of the four is the normal cell line, F111. The F2412 and F1849 produce tumors in the neonatal rat, whereas the F111 and F1706 do not.

The basal and fluoride stimulated levels of adenylate cyclase of each of the four cell lines is compared in Table 1. The only remarkable difference in the values is the elevation of the basal level of the F2412 at 120 hrs. The elevation of the basal values at zero time must be due to the effect of trypsinization or the addition of fresh serum, which is added to inhibit the trypsin, since the zero time values are obtained by trypsinization of 120-hour cultures. Since the fluoride affects ATPase and adenylate cyclase, which are membrane bound enzymes, presumably the chemical carcinogen has altered the membrane of the F2412 cells. Similar elevations are seen in the zero time values for the fluoride stimulated levels of F111, but not F2412. The lowest values for basal and fluoride stimulated levels of adenylate cyclase are found at 18 hours and 48 hours during which time the

4

cells are multiplying most rapidly.

Similarly, the highest values obtained for cyclic AMP (Table 2) in the cell lines were found between 0 and 8 hours after trypsinization of the cells. In general, all of the cyclic AMP values decrease after 8 hours reaching their lowest levels at 168 hours. The F2412 and F1849 cells have the lowest levels of cyclic AMP and this is particularly apparent during logarithmic growth. From comparison of the adenylate cyclase and cyclic AMP levels, it appears that a correlation exists between basal levels of adenylate cyclase and cyclic AMP levels except for the 120-hour value of F2412.

The effects of adding exogenous cyclic AMP or dibutyryl cyclic AMP is generally found to retard the rate of division of cells. Because the cells metabolize the added cyclic AMP to 5' AMP, which may also be inhibitory, inhibition is a consequence of both cyclic AMP and 5' AMP. For this reason, it is best to assay the effect of cyclic AMP on cells at several cell densities. This relation between cell density and cyclic AMP inhibition has been demonstrated by van Wijk, Wicks, and Clay (21). The effects of exogenous cyclic AMP on each of the cell lines is shown in Table 3. The tumor cell line F1849 was not inhibited by cyclic AMP and F2412 was only slightly inhibited, whereas the normal cell lines were markedly inhibited. An explanation for this difference was presented by a previous investigation with WI-38 cells which were also found to be resistant to inhibition by cyclic AMP. This resistance is related to a decreased ability to transport cyclic AMP (22, 23). To test this possibility, each of the four cell lines were incubated in 0.3 mM cyclic AMP for 24 hours and the percent inhibition and cyclic AMP level in each of the cells measured. The results in Table 4 show that there is a correlation between the level of cyclic AMP and the inhibition observed. The tumor cells have considerably lower levels of cyclic AMP than the normals, which suggests a possible mechanism for their resistance to exogenous cyclic AMP. This may be due to a decreased transport of cyclic AMP, or may also result from more rapid destruction by phosphodiesterase.

An attempt to inhibit these tumors in vivo by injection of cyclic AMP would appear futile. However, other agents such as theophylline, the prostaglandins, and dibutyryl cyclic AMP may inhibit the cells. An investigation of the inhibitory effects of these agents is shown in Table 5. Although cyclic AMP does not inhibit the carcinogen or virus transformed cells, theophylline is more inhibitory to these two tumor cells than it is to either of the normal cells. Although dibutyryl cyclic AMP inhibits all four of the cell lines, the addition of equimolar butyrate to the cells is equally inhibitory which probably indicates that the inhibition by dibutyryl cyclic AMP is actually due to the butyrate. The prostaglandin E_1 is more inhibitory to the normal cells than to the tumor cells. The results suggest that theophylline might be more effective than PGE_1 or cyclic AMP in inhibiting the growth of the tumor cells in vivo.

DISCUSSION

The basal adenylate cyclase levels of the 3-methylcholanthrene transformed cell line (F2412) and its cell of origin (F111) are similar except when the cells reach confluency. At confluency the basal level of adenylate cyclase in the F2412 cell line is approximately three times as great as the normal cell. The significance of this increase is difficult to interpret, as the F111 cell line shows a sharp decrease in growth at confluency whereas the F2412 continues to grow and is not density inhibited. To obtain zero time values, cells from confluent cultures were trypsinized. Since this is the only difference in treatment between the 120-hour values and the zero time values for adenylate cyclase, the marked increase in the basal values for this time period must be due to the trypsinization procedure. Although the normal cells show a 7-fold (basal) and 2-fold (fluoride) increase following the trypsinization, the tumor cell (3-MC) is increased only 2-fold in the basal level and in the fluoride level not at all. Effects of trypsin on cell division, cyclic AMP levels, and on membrane phenomenon have been reported. The elevation of adenylate cyclase by trypsinization of normal cells, with slight effect on tumor cells, may also be related to the above phenomena.

6

Some correlation is seen between the levels of adenylate cyclase and cyclic AMP in the cell; for example, the highest cyclic AMP and adenylate cyclase values are found after trypsinization. The cyclic AMP levels in the cells decrease from this point and reach their lowest levels at confluency. The lack of correlation between cyclic AMP and adenylate cyclase values, especially in the F2412 cell line, after the first 48 hours may be due to an increase in phosphodiesterase which has been shown to be an inducible enzyme (24, 25). A rise in phosphodiesterase may lower the cyclic AMP levels in spite of the increase in adenylate cyclase. Although the values for cyclic AMP in the four rat embryo cell lines are similar to those reported by others (3), they are at least 10-fold higher than those that we have found for the 6C3HED, L5178Y, and L1210 tumor cells in vivo and nearly 100 times greater than normal mouse liver and spleen (26). The explanation for these considerable differences is not presently clear. Neither of the tumor cells are inhibited by exogenous cyclic AMP, whereas the normal cells are greatly inhibited. A possible explanation for this difference is the observation of lower cellular levels of cyclic AMP found in the tumor cells after incubation in cyclic AMP. This may be due to a reduced ability of cyclic AMP to be transported by the tumor cells or to higher phosphodiesterase levels in the tumor cells. The inability to effectively transport cyclic AMP may represent the loss of an important control mechanism. Cells at high density, as in tissues, may regulate the rate of cell division of each other by inter and intra-cellular transport of cyclic AMP. Loss of this relationship may permit the tumor cell to grow independently of other cells in the organ without the restraint of cyclic AMP.

SUMMARY

A normal rat embryo cell line was transformed <u>in vitro</u> by 3-methylcholanthrene to a cell which produces tumors in the Fischer rat. The adenylate cyclase, cyclic AMP level during growth in tissue culture and response to exogenous cyclic AMP were investigated. For comparison a high passage rat embryo cell line and a cell line transformed by RLV, arising from the same original cell line were also examined. The carcinogenic transformation results in a cell of smaller cell volume which divides more rapidly. Treatment with trypsin increases the basal level of adenylate cyclase in the normal cell considerably, but alters the adenylate cyclase of the malignant cell only slightly.

The inability of cyclic AMP or dibutyryl cyclic AMP to inhibit the tumor cells is believed to be due to a decreased ability to transport cyclic AMP. This may represent the loss of an important control mechanism in which cells in organized structures control the rate of division of each other.

REFERENCES

1. W. L. Ryan and M. L. Heidrick, Science, 162, 1484 (1968).
2. M. L. Heidrick and W. L. Ryan, Cancer Res., 31, 1313, (1971).
3. M. M. Burger, B. M. Bombik, B. McL. Breckenridge, and J. R. Sheppard, Nature New Biol., 239, 161, (1972).
4. J. Otten, G. S. Johnson, and I. Pastan, J. Biol. Chem. 247, 7082, (1972).
5. J. Otten, J. Bader, G. S. Johnson, and I. Pastan, J. Biol. Chem., 247, 1632 (1972).
6. J. R. Sheppard, Nature New Biol., 236, 14, (1972).
7. B. Weiss, H. M. Shein, and R. Snyder, Life Sciences, 10, 1253 (1971).
8. H. D. Brown, S. K. Chattopadhyay, H. P. Morris, and S. N. Pennington, Cancer Res., 30, 123, (1970).
9. R. R. Burk, Nature, 219, 1272 (1968).
10. F. R. Butcher, D. F. Scott, V. R. Potter, and H. P. Morris, Cancer Res., 32, 2135 (1972).
11. D. O. Allen, J. Munshower, H. P. Morris, and G. Weber, Cancer Res., 31, 557, (1971).
12. C. V. Peery, G. S. Johnson, and I. Pastan, J. Biol. Chem., 246, 5785, (1971).
13. M. H. Makman, Proc. Nat. Acad. Sci., 68, 2127 (1971).
14. R. R. Gantt, J. R. Martin, and V. J. Evans, J. Nat. Cancer Inst., 42, 369 (1969).
15. K. K. Sanford, B. E. Barker, M. W. Woods, R. Parshad, and L. W. Law, J. Nat. Cancer Inst., 39, 705, (1967).
16. A. E. Freeman, P. J. Price, R. J. Bryan, R. J. Gordon, R. V. Gilden, G. J. Kelloff, and R. J. Huebner, Proc. Nat. Acad. Sci., 68, 445, (1971).
17. M. H. Makman, Science, 170, 1421 (1970).
18. G. Krishna, B. Weiss, and B. B. Brodie, J. Pharmacol. Exp. Ther., 163, 379 (1968).
19. G. Brooker, L. J. Thomas, and M. M. Appleman, Biochemistry, 7, 4177, (1968).
20. A. G. Gilman, Proc. Nat. Acad. Sci., 67, 305, (1970).
21. R. van Wijk, W. D. Wicks, and K. Clay, Cancer Res., 32, 1905 (1972).
22. M. L. Heidrick and W. L. Ryan, Cancer Res., 30, 376, (1970).

23. W. L. Ryan and M. A. Durick, Science, 177, 1002, (1972).
24. V. Maganiello and M. Vaughan, Proc. Nat. Acad. Sci., 69, 269 (1972).
25. M. d'Armiento, G. S. Johnson, and I. Pastan, Proc. Nat. Acad. Sci., 69, 459 (1972).
26. W. L. Ryan and J. E. McClurg, Tissue Levels of Cyclic AMP and Tumor Inhibition, Conference on Cyclic AMP and Immune Responses, January 7-10, 1973, (in press).

Table 1

Adenylate Cyclase of Rat Embryo Cell Lines

Basal Level

Time (hours)	F111	F1706	F1849	F2412
0	47.7	13.2	10.2	45.6
18	2.6	3.9	1.3	3.2
48	7.5	7.8	2.3	5.9
120	7.7	8.7	3.4	23.6

Fluoride-Stimulated Level

Time (hours)	F111	F1706	F1849	F2412
0	124.0	43.0	102.0	62.0
18	5.4	11.8	10.3	5.9
48	48.0	29.0	17.0	11.0
120	67.0	59.0	20.0	68.0

Values pmoles cyclic AMP formed/minute/mg. of protein at 30°. Linear rates were obtained for 20 minutes. The 15 minute value was used for the calculations. Values for 0 time obtained by trypsinization of confluent cultures. Logarithmic growth obtained at 18 and 48 hours. Cells were confluent at 120 hours. Cells were plated at a density of $50/mm^2$.

Table 2

Cyclic AMP Level of Rat Embryo Cell Lines During Growth

Hours	F111	F1706	F1849	F2412
0	60	200	336	97
8	102	120	67	43
24	46	84	29	19
48	50	68	18	15
120	34	9	16	16
168	15	3	10	4

Cells were seeded at $50/mm^2$. Values are pmoles/10^6 cells. Average of five determinations. Logarithmic growth occurs at 24 and 48 hours and cells are confluent at 120 hours. To convert pmoles/10^6 cells to pmoles/10^{-1} mg. multiply values by: F111 = 0.42, F1706 = 0.39, F1849 = 0.48, and F2412 = 0.76.

Table 3

Cyclic AMP Inhibition of Rat Embryo Cell Lines

	F2412			F1849	
mM	A	B	mM	A	B
0.3	0	10	0.3	0	0
0.7	18	26	0.7	0	0
1.0	14	28	1.0	0	0

	F1706			F111	
mM	A	B	mM	A	B
0.3	23	48	0.3	14	35
0.7	46	65	0.7	59	65
1.0	57	74	1.0	60	69

Cell density for A = 54 cells/mm^2; B = 27 cells/mm^2. Percent inhibition 72 hours after plating of cells.

11

Table 4

Level of Cyclic AMP in Rat Embryo Cells
After Incubation in Exogenous Cyclic AMP

	Cyclic AMP/10^6 Cells	% Inhibition
F1706	7546	32
F111	5038	20
F1849	3807	0
F2412	2100	0

Cells were plated at a density of 50 cells/mm^2. 0.3 mM cyclic AMP added to each experimental group at the time of plating. Cells were washed six times with cold saline before the addition of perchloric acid. Cyclic AMP levels and percent inhibition determined at 24 hours. Values are an average of four determinations.

Table 5

Response of Rat Embryo Cell Lines to
Theophylline, Dibutyryl Cyclic AMP, Cyclic AMP, and PGE$_1$

Inhibitor	F2412	F1849	F1706	F111
Theophylline, 1 mM	84	75	26	40
Dibutyryl Cyclic AMP, 1 mM	39	53	54	65
Butyrate, 1 mM	39	38	48	68
Cyclic AMP, 1 mM	10	0	65	62
PGE$_1$ 25 µg/ml.	13	0	20	44

Percent inhibition determined after 72 hours incubation. Cells were plated at a density of 50 cells/mm^2.

12

FIGURE 1. ORIGIN AND CHARACTERISTICS OF RAT EMBRYO CELL LINES

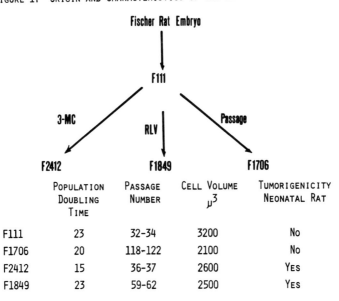

	POPULATION DOUBLING TIME	PASSAGE NUMBER	CELL VOLUME μ^3	TUMORIGENICITY NEONATAL RAT
F111	23	32–34	3200	No
F1706	20	118–122	2100	No
F2412	15	36–37	2600	YES
F1849	23	59–62	2500	YES

DISCUSSION

P. Brown, Wayne University: Did you look at the effect of the cyclic AMP on the naturally occurring nucleotide pools at all?

W. Ryan, University of Nebraska: No, we have not.

T.T. Puck, University of Colorado: I wonder if it wouldn't be worthwhile, if you haven't already done so, to use as a control in every one of these experiments, the identical experiment with theophylline to see what part of the effect is due to the action of phosphodiesterase. Are such experiments with theophylline the experiments to which you were referring when you said the time would not permit you to talk about the effects?

W. Ryan: Well, we've done experiments with theophylline on cells in culture and also experiments in vitro. One of the problems we've had with theophylline is that although it's supposed to inhibit phosphodiesterase, one would therefore expect that it would increase the cyclic AMP levels in the cell. We have seen no increase in cyclic AMP in tissues as a result of using theophylline.

R. Sharma, V.A. Hospital, Memphis: I would like to comment about caffeine and theophylline. We have done some work with caffeine in adrenal hormone tissues, where caffeine is used to increase cyclic AMP level by blocking phosphodiesterase, but we find that the hormone response has actually decreased. At this time, we had not measured cyclic AMP, but we would have expected that it should increase if caffeine does raise cyclic AMP level.

14

T.T. Puck: I would like to remind everyone that some
of these equilibrium responses are extremely rapid.
Dr. Abraham Hsie has studied some of them while he was
still with us at the University of Colorado. You might easily
get changes in the amount of cyclase activity secondarily
to treatment with theophylline or other substances, so
that one has to interpret experiments with great care.

R. Johnson, Vanderbilt University: It is fairly well
known that theophylline can inhibit adenylate cyclase
and this can complicate the interpretation of results. However,
Dr. J. Beavo, of the University of California at Davis, some
time ago found numbers of other methyl xanthine derivatives
which inhibit phosophodiesterase with relatively different
potentials. One of these, which is about twenty times more
potent than theophylline is 1-methyl-3-isobutyl xanthine.
We have found that it is very effective in increasing cyclic
AMP levels in cultured HeLa cells.

G. Weber, Indiana Univeristy: I think that it is a rather
important the cyclic AMP levels did not relate to the growth
in malignancy of the tumors. This brings up a question.
How was the cyclic AMP measured? Has compartmentation
of cyclic AMP in the cells been taken into consideration?
The reason I am asking this is because the total cyclic AMP
might not be the important part, the important part may
be the membrane. The nucleolar cyclic AMP may be the
important factor. The second question, you referred to
cyclic AMP inhibition throughout. Was this cyclic AMP
or was it the dibutyryl derivative, or some other factor?
Third question: you said that theophylline did not have
an effect under these circumstances. The concentration
of theophylline may matter. It requires rather high concentrations, so that it would be interesting for us to know what
concentration you used.

W. Ryan: I don't know whether or not cyclic AMP
is compartmented. I think that's an important question
if we can find a way to answer it. The assays were done

15

by Gilman's procedure; we prepared the samples by Brooker's technique. The theophylline concentrations that we have used are 1 millimolar. Throughout these experiments we used cyclic AMP, not dibutyryl cyclic AMP. We've had problems with dibutyryl cyclic AMP. Our experiments suggest that the tumor cells are inhibited with dibutyryl cyclic AMP, but if one runs butyric acid controls at the same molar concentration, one gets as much inhibition as obtained with the dibutyryl cyclic AMP. That may not be a fair control, but it's enough to bother me about trying to interpret what the data mean.

T.T. Puck: I'm glad you are introducing this matter of butyrated cells. It's a complex problem and I suspect that Dr. Weber has some more to say about that.

G. Weber: The reason I brought up this question is precisely because of the answers you have given. The theophylline concentration is probably too low and perhaps papaverine would have been better. The reason I brought up the dibutyryl derivitive is because we have observed that butyric acid can be frequently as inhibitory as dibutyryl cyclic AMP. It inhibits hexokinase and glucokinase and interferes with various other cell responses. This might be of interest to most of us.

T.T. Puck: Do you have any idea about the mechanism of action of the butyrate? We have found that not only butyrate but valyrate and other acids mimic this effect.

G. Weber: This is under investigation, but we reported earlier that the addition of free fatty acids inhibits various glycolytic enzymes. They can block glycolysis in a dose dependent and time dependent fashion.

I. Pastan, National Institutes of Health: The effect of 1 millimolar theophylline in a few different cell lines has been studied by Dr. D'Armiento in our laboratory. Generally, it increases cyclic AMP levels about 26 fold.

W. Ryan: I'd like to ask Dr. Pastan at what time did you measure the cyclic AMP levels?

I. Pastan: We usually measured cyclic AMP levels initially at 15 minutes and 30 minutes after the addition of theophylline. I do not remember how long the effects lasts, however.

T.T. Puck: I think one has to keep in mind here that different cells might very well respond in markedly different ways, that the central nature of the action of cyclic AMP appears to be to modulate and demodulate by a variety of different metabolic processes.

J.J. Kowal, University Hospital: I agree with you. In the adrenal tumor cells we found that levels of theophylline which were capable of increasing steroid synthesis did not significantly increase endogenous or exogenous secretion of cyclic AMP. Secondly, in terms of phosphodiesterase inhibitors, another word of caution: papaverine seems to be an excellent inhibitor of site 1 oxidative phosphorylation and can slow down cells just on that basis. One cannot really isolate that effect from other effects without considering this fact.

M. Chasin, Squibb Institute for Medical Research: When you measured cyclic AMP in these cells which could have exogenous cyclic AMP, was cyclic AMP just in the cells or was it measured in the cells plus the medium?

W. Ryan: In no case was the medium present, although when we started these experiments we washed the cells with saline because Otten, Johnson and Paston (ref. 4) published a paper describing the effects of washing the cells on the levels of cyclic AMP. In all the remainder of the experiments, what we did was simply to pour off the medium without washing. We really haven't seen much difference whether the cells are washed or not washed, but I suspect that if one is going to wash them with cold saline to remove any medium before cyclic AMP measurements start, that this washing has to be done quite carefully.

METABOLISM OF CYCLIC AMP IN

NORMAL AND TRANSFORMED FIBROBLASTS

J. R. Sheppard*, R. Cromwell,
R. Meyers, and W. J. McLaughlin
Division of Neurology,
University of Colorado Medical School
Denver, Colorado

Abstract: The activities of the enzymes which catalyze
the synthesis and degradation of cyclic AMP in
cultured mouse fibroblasts have been studied. A
comparison of the normal, contact-inhibited cells
with spontaneous and virus transformed cells indicates that the transformed cell lines have higher
specific activities of both synthetic and degradative
enzymes. An attempt to reconcile these differences
in enzyme specific activity with those of a previous
study concerning the basal levels of cyclic AMP in
normal and transformed cells is made and discussed.
A more thorough kinetic analysis of the cyclic nucleotide phosphodiesterase activity shows little variation
of the kinetic parameters and suggests that differen-

*Present address: Dight Institute
                  Botany Bldg., Univ. of Minnesota
                  Minneapolis, Minnesota 55455

19

ces in the absolute quantity of the enzyme or an activator may account for the difference observed in specific activity between normal and transformed cells.

INTRODUCTION

Dibutyryl cyclic AMP has been shown to inhibit the growth of transformed mouse fibroblasts growing in culture (1). Subsequent studies have shown that cyclic AMP levels are lower in transformed cells when compared to the parent, contact-inhibited, normally growing cells (2). The studies presented here concerning the enzymes responsible for synthesis and breakdown of cyclic AMP, were started in the hope of determining a possible enzymic basis for the depressed cyclic AMP levels observed in the transformed cells. These studies were initially presented at the Fifth International Congress of Pharmacology 1972.

METHODS

Conditions for the growth of the mouse fibroblasts have been previously published (1). The cells were a gift of Drs. H. Green and R. Pollack and were routinely tested for possible mycoplasma contamination in our laboratory.

Preparation of cells for enzyme assay

Confluent cultures were harvested by scraping the cells from disposable Bellco roller bottles after all but 20 ml of the medium had been removed. The cells were then pelleted at 1500 rpm in a Sorvall table top centrifuge for 15 minutes, then washed twice with 0.32M sucrose in 50 mM tris, pH 7.5 at 4°. All subsequent steps were also done at 4°. The final washed pellet was resuspended in 2 ml. of the sucrose-tris buffer and this suspension homogenized for 60 seconds in a Polytron homogenizer at setting 5. This homogenate was used for the assay of both adenylate cyclase and phosphodiesterase.

Enzyme Assays:

The adenylate cyclase assay was patterned after the method of Krishna et al (3) as modified by Perkins and Moore (4). A typical assay incubation mixture contained 0.05 ml of 0.014M cyclic AMP in 0.025 M Tris-HCl, pH 7.5; 0.4 ml of buffer solution containing 0.10 M Tris HCl. pH 7.5 and 25 mM theophylline and 12.5 mM Mg S04 and 12.5 mM KCl; 0.1 ml of 25 mM Phosphoenol-pyruvate in 25 mM Tris HCL pH 7.5 (from Sigma); 0.02 ml pyruvate kinase (2.0 mg/ml in water, from Sigma); 0.05 ml dithiothrietol (20 mM, from Sigma); 0.05 ml of 8 mM ATP in 0.25 M tris-HCL pH 7.5 containing 1.4 x 10^6 cpm of ^{3}H ATP (15 c/mM from New England Nuclear), approximately 2-400 ug protein in 0.2 ml of homogenizing buffer (other additives when needed), and water to bring the volume to 1.0 ml. Assays were started with the addition of the substrate solution and incubated at 30° for 20 minutes in a water shaker.

The phosphodiesterase assay was that of O'Dea et al (5) using the Amberlite SB-2 ion exchange paper from Reeve-Angel. The ^{3}H-Cyclic AMP was purchased from New England Nuclear. The Gilman cyclic AMP assay (6) was used and specifics concerning the procedure are published elsewhere (2). Protein was measured by the method of Lowry et al (7). The phosphodiesterase in-hibitor R 020 was the kind gift of Dr. H. Sheppard at Hoffman La-Roche, Nutley, New Jersey.

RESULTS

Adenylate Cyclase

The formation of cyclic AMP using homogenates

21

prepared for both normal and transformed cells is
linear with respect to protein concentration up to at
least 1.0 mg. protein per reaction tube. Linearity is
also observed with respect to time up to 30 min. of
incubation. The pH optima of the assay was observed
over the range 7.5 to 8.0 and was similar for all lines
tested. A comparison of the specific activity of the
adenylate cyclase from normal and transformed cell
lines is shown in Table 1. Both spontaneous (3T6) and
virus transformed (py 3T3) cells have significantly
higher specific activities in relation to the normal 3T3
cell line. Fluoride, which is thought to specifically
stimulate the catalytic subunit of the enzyme, gives a
proportional increase to the basal activity level of the
cell lines tested (about three fold). Prostaglandin E_1 (a
gift from Dr. J. Pike of the Upjohn Co.) which has been
suggested to stimulate the receptor subunit of adenylate
cyclase was observed to increase the activity of the 3T3
and Py3T3 homogenates about two fold but only 50%
stimulation occurred with the 3T6 cell line.

Table 1

Adenylate Cyclase Specific Activity

of Homogenates of Normal and Transformed Cells

Cell Type	p moles of cAMP formed min/mg prot		
	Basal	F⁻ (8mM)	PGE_1 (10 µg/ml)
3T3	6+2	20+ 4	10+3
py3T3	12+4	38+ 7	29+6
3T6	32+7	94+11	49+7

PHOSPHODIESTERASE:

The hydrolysis of cyclic AMP to 5' AMP is linear under the conditions studied up to 20 minues of incubation and 400 μg of protein per assay. The pH optima of the various cell lines are shown in Table 2. The 3T3 cell line has an optimum of activity at pH 7.5 whereas the transformed lines exhibit an optimum at pH 8.0.

Table 2

cAMP Phosphodiesterase pH Optima

in Normal and Transformed Cells

Cell Type	pH Optima
3T3	7.0 - 7.5
py3T3	8.0
3T6	8.0

Specific activity of the transformed lines under optimal, non-limiting conditions shows that the transformed lines have approximately twice the activity of the normal 3T3 line. Kinetic analysis using the Lineweaver-Burk reciprocal plot indicates that the normal and transformed lines have similar apparent low Km constants (Table 3). The high Km constant was not studied. Inhibition of the phosphodiesterase from different sources by theophylline, papaverine or RO 20 also show similarities. Figures 1 and 2 are some of the data from these studies. Although Figure 2 might be interpreted as evidence for some kinetic variation, we do not feel the differences are significant.

Table 3

Kinetic Studies of cAMP Phosphodiesterase

in Normal and Transformed Cells

Cell Type	Vmax (p moles cAMP Degraded) (mg prot/min)	Km(μM)
3T3	3.0 ± 0.5	1.0
py3T3	6.8 ± 0.6	1.2
3T6	5.5 ± 1.4	1.0

As a measure of the phosphodiesterase activity in the whole cell and also for an estimate of the turnover of cyclic AMP in the various cell lines, we measured the cellular levels of cyclic AMP after exposure of the cells, as they grew in culture, to papaverine. Table 4 shows that a large difference is observable between the normal and transformed cells. Both transformed lines have an immediate and large increase in their cyclic AMP level but the normal 3T3 line has no such effect resulting from exposure to papaverine.

Table 4

Effect of Papaverine on cAMP Levels in

Normal and Transformed Cells

Cell type	cAMP (p-moles/mg prot) time after exposure to 10^{-4} M papaverine		
	0	15'	180'
3T3	24+3	25+3	28+4
py3T3	14+2	113+12	57+6
3T6	12+2	46+7	20+4

DISCUSSION

Previous studies have shown that transformed cells have a depressed level of cyclic AMP in comparison to the normal, contact-inhibited cells (2, 8). The studies reported here concerning cyclic nucleotide phosphodiesterase could conceivably explain the difference. However, the observation that transformed cells also have increased activities of adenylate cyclase suggests several different interpretations of the data presented here: 1. That phosphodiesterase is the more important factor in the maintenance of cyclic AMP level. 2. That other factors not studied or discussed here may be also important. 3. That the assays used here are not valid reflections of the enzymes activities as they exist in the whole cell.

Perry et al (9) have also looked at the activity of adenylate cyclase in normal and transformed mouse fibroblasts and our results are comparable with regard to basal activities but their study showed more sensitivity of their enzyme to prostaglandin. Possibly their preparation of the enzyme, which differed from ours, has an effect on this parameter. Weiss et al (10) have studied adenylate cyclase and phosphodiesterase of normal and SV40 transformed astrocytes from newborn hamster brains. These authors showed a decreased activity of adenylate cyclase in the virus transformed line and no difference with regard to phosphodiesterase activity. Similar studies by Bürk(11) also showed a decreased activity of adenylate cyclase in the polyoma transformed BHK cells compared to the parent BHK cell line. Looking at all of these studies, no distinct pattern is perceived.

The experiment which studied cyclic AMP levels in whole cells after exposure to papaverine, although further suggesting that adenylate cyclase activity may be increased in transformed cells or that turnover of cyclic

Inhibition Studies of Py, 3T3, 3T6, and SV Cell Homogenates with Theophylline

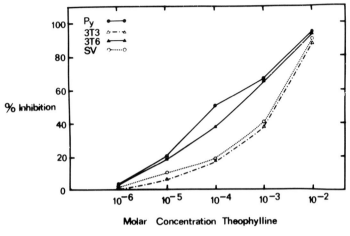

Figure 1

Inhibition Studies of Py, 3T3, 3T6, and SV Cell Homogenates with Papaverine

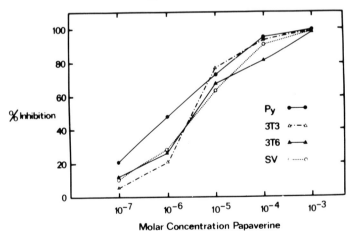

Figure 2

AMP occurs at a faster rate in transformed cells is also suspect to artifact. The transport of papaverine into the transformed cell may be facilitated by the membrane changes known to exist in the transformed cell membrane (12). Increased transport of the inhibitor would lead to increased inhibition of phosphodiesterase leading to elevated cyclic AMP levels.

In summary, differences are observed to occur in the specific activities of the enzymes catalyzing synthesis and degradation of cyclic AMP in normal and transformed mouse fibroblasts. The importance of these observations with regard to cellular levels of cyclic AMP and their possible use in the control of cell proliferation are open to conjecture and further study.

ACKNOWLEDGMENTS

The excellent technical assistance of Ms. Doris Gaskin is appreciated. These studies were conducted with the support of the American Cancer Society (BC-68) and the Damon Runyon Foundation (1161).

REFERENCES

1. Sheppard, J.R., Proc. Nat. Acad. Sci., U.S., 68, 1316, 1971
2. Sheppard, J.R., Nature New Biol., 236, 14, 1972
3. Krishna, G., Weiss, B., Brodie, S.B., J. Pharmacol. Exp. Ther., 163, 379, 1968
4. Perkins, J.R., Moore, M., J. Biol. Chem., 246 62, 1971
5. O'Dea, R.F., Haddox, M.K., Goldberg, N.D., J. Biol. Chem., 246, 6183, 1971
6. Gilman, A.G., Proc. US Nat. Acad. Sci., 67, 305, 1970
7. Lowry, O.H., Rosebrough, N.J., Farr, A.L., and Randall, R.J., J.Biol. Chem., 188, 265 (1951)

8. Sheppard, J.R. and Lehman, J.M., in Medical Aspects of Cyclic AMP and Prostaglandins, ed. R. Kahn, Academic Press, 1972
9. Perry, C.V., Johnson, G.S., Pastan, I., J. Biol. Chem., <u>246</u>, 5785, 1971
10. Weiss, B., Shein, H.M., Snyder, R., Life Sciences, <u>10</u>, 1253, 1971
11. Bürk, R. R., Nature, <u>219</u>, 1272, 1968

12. Burger, M.M., in "Current topics in cellular regulation" (B. L. Horecker, ed.), Vol. 3, p 135 Academic Press, 1971

DISCUSSION

T.T. Puck, University of Colorado: In opening Dr. Sheppard's paper for discussion, I would like to propose that we keep in mind the fact that the role of cyclic AMP on cell growth will be a continuing theme throughout this Symposium. Therefore, let's not try to solve all of the problems involved in a single discussion, but rather reconsider issues presented in successive papers in light of the new data presented in each paper.

C. Zeilig, Vanderbilt University: I'd like to say that we've been studying the regulation of growth in HeLa cells. We found that dibutyryl cyclic AMP could inhibit the growth of HeLa cells. We also found that sodium butyrate and 5' AMP could inhibit cell proliferation. When we analyzed DNA content of HeLa cells, which were completely inhibited after three days of treatment with dibutyryl cyclic AMP, in the hope of getting an idea of where in the cell cycle they were stopped, we found DNA contents exactly equal to control logarithmic HeLa cells. The same result has recently been reported by Van Wijk and Wicks. There are several possible interpretations of that result, but the one that we favored at the time and continue to favor is that the cells were stopped in their original positions in the cell cycle in the same proportions as the untreated cells, the same interpretation that you have made.

J.R. Sheppard, University of Colorado: May I ask you just after the fact, were you studying cells that had been completely stopped in their reproduction or just slowed down?

C. Zeilig: Completely stopped.

J.R. Sheppard: I should comment on the other nucleotides which we used as controls. We have looked at butyrate in concentrations five times that of which we were using with the dibutyryl cyclic AMP, and we did not see any effect of butyrate on the growth of these cells. However, Dr. Prasad, who has studied the neuroblastoma, has seen some effect of butyrate on the growth of these cells in the culture, and interestingly, together, we have observed an elevation of the endogenous level of cyclic AMP after exposure of neuroblastoma to butyrate.

E.E. Smith, Boston University School of Medicine: The previous speaker indicated that trypsinization increased cyclic AMP levels. Did I get that impression from him?

J.R. Sheppard: In our hands, trypsinization leads to an immediate depression of cyclic AMP within 15 seconds.

E.E. Smith: This is what I thought, too, but it seems as if Dr. Ryan indicated there was an increase. Is this true?

W. Ryan, University of Nebraska: I don't think we really have any disagreement. If you notice the time period over which Dr. Sheppard measured cyclic AMP, what he saw was the decrease within a relatively short period of time, like 10 to 15 minutes.

J.R. Sheppard: Yes. That is true, with 10 to 15 minutes.

W. Ryan: Then the cyclic AMP level went back up. What I suggested was that perhaps in our studies what we were seeing, since we used much longer periods of time in which to measure the cyclic AMP, was just the increase which shown after that initial decrease.

J.R. Sheppard: We didn't see any appreciable increase above the normal basal level.

T.T. Puck: I want to remind us again that the cell specificities are important. We cannot expect to have these various phenomena repeated exactly from cell to cell. If we can see trends or similar directions of change, this may be all that we hope for at this state of ignorance about the molecular bases of the changes described.

R.W. Longton, NMRI, NNMC: Your statement on nutrient effects in relation to cyclic AMP levels is of interest to me. Dr. J. S. Cole III and I have observed the effect of 1 millimolar aspartic acid on the inhibition of cellular growth in Minneapolis esophageal epithelial cells (MEE) and in human embryonic brain cells (HEB). The results that you showed and those which Dr. Pastan observed on the effect of dibutyryl cyclic AMP inhibition of cellular growth, we also observed with the 1 millimolar aspartic acid, so your statement was rather interesting.

J.R. Sheppard: The implication being that aspartate would somehow interfere with nutrient transport?

R.W. Longton: It appears to have a relationship to the cyclic AMP levels by metabolic effects. We haven't measured the cyclic AMP levels at this point. We have intended to do this and I have discussed this previously with Dr. Pastan.

B. Weiss, Medical College of Pennsylvania: I would like to propose a possible explanation for some of the results that you and Dr. Ryan obtained with the phosphodiesterase inhibitors. It is now well established that there are multiple forms of phosphodiesterase in tissues. For example, we have found that there are six molecular forms of the enzyme in rat cerebellum. More recently we have studied the multiple forms of phosphodiesterase in various cloned tumor cell lines, including astrocytoma cell lines and neuroblastoma cell lines. Each tumor tissue has a distinct pattern of phosphodiesterase activity. Moreover, we found each form of phosphodiesterase can be inhibited differentially by different drugs. For example, theophylline preferentially inhibited one of the forms of phosphodiesterase, whereas other phosphodiesterase inhibitors, such as papaverine and trifluoroperazine, differentially inhibit other forms of the enzyme. Therefore, your studies showing that papaverine, for example, increased the level of cyclic AMP in tumor tissue and not in normal tissue, may result in the differences in the types of phosphodiesterases that may exist in normal and tumor tissues. I think one is really compelled now to study the different forms of phosphodiesterase in the different types of tissues, and to determine which inhibitor antagonizes the activity of each of the forms of phosphodiesterase. That inhibitor should raise the concentration of cyclic AMP in that cell.

J.R. Sheppard: We have observed two different types of phosphodiesterase, one with a low Km and one with a higher binding constant in all our cell lines and we've concentrated our studies on the low Km enzyme. There may be some substance to the suggestion that there may be differences between normal and transformed cells insofar as the phosphodiesterase isoenzymes.

G. Weber, Indiana University: I think the question of the different isozymic forms of phosphodiesterase is a highly relevant one. A paper will appear by Clark, Morris and Weber in the February issue of Cancer Research related to this fact. I will also refer to this in my lecture this afternoon. There is an isozyme shift in the hepatomas that relates to the growth rate of these tumors. Accordingly, an enzyme emerges that has a higher affinity to cyclic AMP in the rapidly growing tumors, so the overall measurements of phosphodiesterase activity, as this comment suggested, eventually will have to be replaced by the measure of the isoenzymes. Moreover, the phosphodiesterase assay is usually done in total homogenates or rather in the super-

natant fluid, because most of it is supposed to be there.
But what may matter is the phosphodiesterase at the same
location as the cyclase, in the membrane, and I think you
will hear a report regarding this from both Dr. Tomasi
and Dr. Réthy later on in this symposium.

G. Cherayil, Medical College of Wisconsin: I am a
novice in the study of the metabolism of cyclic AMP, but
I would like to ask what could we expect during the treatment
of these cells with trypsin. Don't we expect the enzymes
involved in the metabolism of cyclic AMP to be affected by
trypsin treatment, for example, the adenyl cyclase or phosphodiesterase?

J.R. Sheppard: The effect of trypsin on phosphodiesterase, has been studied by other laboratories. Dr. Cheung's
comes to mind. Trypsin stimulates in vitro preparations
of phosphodiesterase. This possibility occurred to us,
but in cells that had been treated with trypsin, we have
not observed any increased activities of phosphodiesterase
in homogenates. What happens if one takes phosphodiesterase
in pure form and then treats it with trypsin? There is a
stimulation. One paradoxical thing that we have observed
was that although we get a depression of cellular cyclic
AMP level after exposure of cells to trypsin, we actually
get an activation of cyclase activity. This is the same
thing that Dr. Ryan has shown in his presentation. The
same thing appears to have occurred in the synchronized
population. Mackman has shown that synchronized cells
have an elevated activity of adenylate cyclase during mitosis
just at the same time we see a depression of cyclate AMP.
These observations are paradoxical.

M. Blecher, Georgetown University: I'd like to offer
a word of caution to those of you who are using dibutyryl
cyclic AMP to mimic the action of cyclic AMP for inhibiting
the growth of cells, and who are thereafter using butyrate
in an attempt to determine whether the effect of dibutyryl
cyclic AMP is indeed due to its butyrate content. The reason

for this is that undoubtedly you are aware you are using
butyrate at concentrations similar to those of the dibutyryl
cyclate AMP. In the absence of any additional information
this makes sense to do. However, we have recently published
the results of investigations of the catabolism of the two
monobutyryl cyclate AMPs and the dibutyryl cyclic AMP
in extracts of five rat tissues. We have found that N^6-amidohy-
drolases and $O^{2'}$-esterases indeed exist for the removal
of the butyryl groups, but these deacylases are rather
weak. They are similar in activity to each other, but are
two orders of magnitude weaker than the corresponding
phosphodiesterase or the 5' nucleotidases. Therefore, the
amounts of butyrate that may be produced from your dibutyryl
cyclic AMP will be rather small, relative to the originally
high concentration of the substrate. They will become
significant only after perhaps days of incubation, but
for short term experiments, the amounts of butyrate produced
enzymatically will be rather negligible and certainly
not nearly that of the initial concentrations of dibutyryl
cyclic AMP with which you are starting. Furthermore,
since we have observed little deacylation of dibutyryl cyclic
AMP by isolated fat cells, one must first establish with
cells in culture that significant deacylation of mono or dibutyryl cyclate AMP can occur before entertaining the possibility
that effects are due to butyrate.

J. Miller, ICN Nucleic Acid Research Institute:
Apparently the active form of dibutyryl cyclic AMP is N^6-
monobutyryl cyclic AMP, so any action that you see of dibutyryl cyclic AMP is going to have to be caused by some esterase
activity. For example, if you need 4 μM N^6-monobutyryl
cyclic AMP to see the action, then you're going to have
to have 4 μM butyrate also formed.

J.R. Sheppard: The most appropriate control was
to use other dibutyryl cyclic nucleotides. We have seen
very little effect of dibutyryl cyclic GMP, suggesting that
butyrate has little effect.

34

J. Miller: I would suggest that people try the N^6-monobutyryl derivative.

T.T. Puck: Well, we have done so and we get virtually identical results with it as with dibutyryl cyclic AMP. Moreover, we can mimic the effects of the dibutyryl compound by using the combination of cyclic AMP and theophylline. So, while this does not rule out completely a supporting role of butyrate, it would seem to show that the cyclic AMP part of the molecule is active.

J.R. Sheppard: We've seen in whole extracts that the removal of the 2' butyrate is fairly rapid. and removal of the N^6-buterate is very slow. You can really eliminate the butyrate problem by using the N^6 monobutyrates.

J. Miller: In a case where you treated with trypsin or insulin, and saw a depression of cyclic AMP levels, did you mention that you saw a transient decrease in cyclic AMP? As the cells increase in number again and then level off, what would the corresponding change in time of cyclic AMP level be? Did it increase before cell growth stopped or did it increase concomitantly as the cell number increased?

J.R. Sheppard: Well, the total amount of cyclic AMP would follow the same contour of the curve. The amount of cyclic AMP per cell would be constant. That is, there would be no change in the basal level of cyclic AMP after the cells had grown to the higher density.

P.A. Galand, Free University of Brussels: You observed that the cells are blocked in a phase of the cell cycle, but when you deal with G_1 phase in fact you deal with what represents 80% of the cell cycle, so it's not so well defined to say that they are blocked in G_1. I would like to ask you what happens when you remove dibutyrate, for example, or any blocking agent you used and follow the kinetic aspect. What do the cells do first? Do they enter first S phase or go into mitosis, or do they enter into some other phase of the cell cycle?

J.R. Sheppard: We have done these experiments and what we see is that there does appear to be some buildup in the G_1 phase but immediately after the removal of the cyclic or dibutyryl cyclic AMP, we can get an increased incorporation into tritiated thymidine, suggesting that some of the cells were stopped in the S phase. Now, when you do this with normal, contact inhibited cells, we see very little thymidine incorporation until about 18 hours after replating or exposure to trypsin.

P.A. Galand: You have no indication on the number of labelled cells, labelled into DNA?

J.R. Sheppard: We've done autoradiography on these cells and it's about 15% of the cells. These are the dibutyryl cyclic AMP treated 3T6 cells. About 15% of the cells continued to incorporate ^{3}H-thymidine.

P.A. Galand: Yes, and what mitotic index as compared with labelling index did you find?

J.R. Sheppard: Normally the mitotic index is about 5% and about 30 hours thereafter we get about 10%, so there is some synchronization in G_1.

G. Krishna, National Institutes of Health: I want to ask if you have ever tried to make measurements of turnover of cyclic AMP instead of measuring steady state levels of cyclic AMP, or of the activities of cyclases and phosphodiesterases? You attempted to measure turnover in the experiment using papaverine as the inhibitor. Probably this may not be the best method, but you can get a better idea by measuring the turnover rates of cyclic AMP in these cells, rather than just a steady state level alone. Have you done any post-labelling studies with ^{32}P or ^{3}H-adenine?

J.R. Sheppard: No, we have not done these studies, but that's a very good suggestion. That's the appropriate way to go about it.

REGULATION OF CELL FUNCTIONS IN FIBROBLASTS BY CYCLIC AMP

GEORGE S. JOHNSON
Laboratory of Molecular Biology
National Institutes of Health, National Cancer Institute

Abstract: Cyclic AMP regulates a variety of functions in normal cells. It controls cell motility, adhesion to the substratum, morphology, growth, and synthesis of mucopolysaccharides. Transformed cells have low cyclic AMP levels. Treatment of transformed cells with Bt_2cAMP restores many aspects of metabolism and behavior towards normal.

INTRODUCTION

Cultured fibroblasts display various growth and behavioral characteristics. They attach to the substratum and migrate across it and assume a characteristic flattened and elongated morphology. The cells increase in number until a critical density is reached when growth ceases. This has been termed "contact or density dependent inhibition of growth". Also, macromolecules such as collagen and mucopolysaccharide are synthesized. Since abnormalities in these properties are usually associated with transformation, a common regulatory mechanism could be altered. Considering the important and ubiquitous nature of the nucleotide adenosine 3',5'-monophosphate (cyclic AMP) it seemed reasonable to us at the start of this study that cyclic AMP could be involved in the regulation of these properties and that cyclic AMP levels could be low in transformed cells.

MOTION AND MORPHOLOGY

We began our studies by the addition of an analog of cyclic AMP, N^6,O^2-dibutyryl cyclic AMP (Bt_2cAMP) to the growth medium of the transformed cells. Cyclic AMP itself was relatively ineffective presumably due to poor penetration into the cell or a more rapid metabolism. We found that cells treated with Bt_2cAMP acquired some of the properties of normal cells; they became more elongated flattened, and often assumed a parallel orientation (1, 2, 3). It should be emphasized that $(bt)_2cAMP$ also had effects on the morphology of untransformed cells; they became even more flattened and elongated (3).

We then used time lapse cinematography to study in more detail the effects of Bt_2cAMP on L-929 cells (4). Several conclusions were drawn from this study. Within 20 minutes after the addition of Bt_2cAMP the cells had a decreased migration across the substratum. Earlier times could not be tested for technical reasons. After a few hours the cells began to elongate and long narrow processes were apparent.

We also studied how rapidly the cells reverted to the morphology of control cells after Bt_2cAMP removal. Within a few minutes, the cells withdrew the narrow processes and began to move about rapidly (4). It should be noted that shortly after removal of the Bt_2cAMP considerable mitotic activity was apparent. This indicates that Bt_2cAMP causes some synchronization of cells in G_2 phase. This is consistent with observation of Willingham et al. in 3T3 cells (5) and Smets in SV40 transformed 3T3 cells (6).

ADHESION TO SUBSTRATUM

In other experiments, cells treated with Bt_2cAMP were shown to adhere more tightly to the substratum (7). This increased adhesion was rapidly initiated, insensitive to cycloheximide and, like the effects on motion and morphology, rapidly reversed when Bt_2cAMP was removed.

LOGARITHMIC GROWTH

The concentration of cyclic AMP within the cell controls the growth rate of cells. Otten et al. (8) reported that there is an inverse correlation between the growth rate and the endogenous levels of cyclic AMP. Cells with low amounts of cyclic AMP grew more rapidly than those with larger amounts. Elevation of cyclic AMP levels in L-929 cells by prostaglandin E_1 (PGE_1) (9) decreased the growth rate (10). PGE_1 failed to elevate cyclic AMP levels in one clone of SV40 transformed 3T3 cells (9). With this line PGE_1 did not inhibit growth (11). Also $(bt)_2cAMP$ decreased the growth rate of several cell lines. This inhibition of growth was potentiated by theophylline, an inhibitor of phosphodiesterase (3).

CONTACT INHIBITION OF GROWTH

Normal embryo cells usually divide until confluency. At this time, growth ceases or continues at a markedly decreased rate. Transformed cells classically do not cease growth at the saturation density of their parent cells but grow to much higher densities. The mechanism for this cessation of growth is not clear. However, the involvement of a "messenger signal" at the membrane during cell contact which then migrates into the nucleus has been proposed. Recent evidenc indicates that cyclic AMP is this messenger. Addition of Bt_2cAMP will decrease the logarithmic growth rate and the saturation density of contact inhibited 3T3 cells (3). Moreover, the intracellular levels of cyclic AMP rise as growth ceases in 3T3 cells and in other contact inhibited cell lines (7, 8), but not in cell lines which do not show contact inhibition of growth. This suggests that an inability to elevate cyclic AMP levels at confluency results in overgrowth. However it doesn't appear to be as simple as this, since the addition of Bt_2cAMP to transformed cells doesn't restore contact inhibition of growth (3). This is contrary to the results reported by Sheppard (12), but agrees with a recent study by Paul (13).

INVOLVEMENT OF MICROTUBULAR PROTEINS

Cells treated with Bt_2cAMP have long narrow processes and also flatten and have a "web-like" appearance (1, 2, 3). (Figures 1 and 2). Colchicine, an inhibitor of microtubular protein polymerization will block this response to Bt_2cAMP (2, 14). Figures 3 and 4 show the effects of cytochalasin B on control and $(bt)_2cAMP$ treated 3T3 cells. Cytochalasin is a drug which is thought to disrupt microfilaments. With this treatment the cells retain the flattened appearance and structures of probable microtubular proteins are clearly visable.

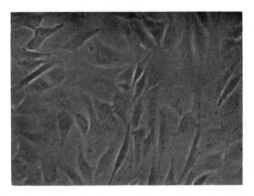

Fig. 1. Morphology of confluent 3T3 cells. Cells were grown as previously described (3). Phase contrast x 160.

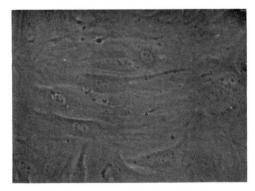

Fig. 2. Morphology of confluent 3T3 cells treated with 1.2 mM $(bt)_2cAMP$. Phase contrast x 160.

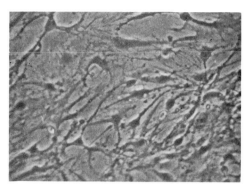

Fig. 3. Effect of cytochalasin B on morphology of 3T3 cells. Cells were incubated with 5 μg/ml cytochalasin B for 30 min at 37°. Phase contrast x 190.

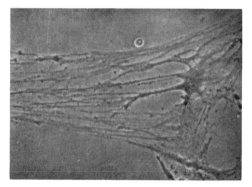

Fig. 4. Effect of cytochalasin B on morphology of 3T3 cells previously treated with 1.2 mM $(bt)_2$cAMP. Cells were incubated with 5 μg/ml cytochalasin B for 30 min at 37°. Phase contrast x 190.

SYNTHESIS OF ACID MUCOPOLYSACCHARIDES

Transformed 3T3 cells secrete less acid mucopolysaccharide than do the parent cells (Tables 1 and 2). Incubation of the cells with Bt_2cAMP plus theophylline results in a pronounced increase in the synthesis by the transformed cells and a smaller increase in the amount of synthesis by the parent 3T3 cells (15). A comparison of the relative amounts synthesized show that the transformed cells synthesize 25% of the amount synthesized by the 3T3 cells and the amount is increased to 85% by Bt_2cAMP treatment (Table 2).

TABLE 1

Sulfated acid mucopolysaccharide production by 3T3 and SV40 transformed 3T3 cells*

Cell line	Sulfate incorporation $cpmX10^{-3}$/mg protein	Ratio
3T3		
Control	444	
Treated	660	1.5
SV40/3T3		
Control	105	
Treated	371	3.5

*Data taken from Reference 15.

TABLE 2

Comparison of amount of sulfated acid mucopolysaccharides produced to that produced by control 3T3 cells

Cell line	Ratio
$\dfrac{\text{SV40/3T3 Control}}{\text{3T3 Control}}$	0.25
$\dfrac{\text{SV40/3T3 Treated}}{\text{3T3 Control}}$	0.85

REFERENCES

(1) G. S. Johnson, R. M. Friedman and I. Pastan, Ann. N. Y. Acad. Sci., 85 (1971) 413.

(2) G. S. Johnson, R. M. Friedman and I. Pastan, Proc. Nat. Acad. Sci., U.S.A., 68 (1971) 425.

(3) G. S. Johnson and I. Pastan, J. Nat. Cancer Inst., 48 (1972) 1377.

(4) G. S. Johnson and I. Pastan, Nature, 235 (1972) 54.

(5) M. C. Willingham, G. S. Johnson and I. Pastan, Biochem. Biophys. Res. Commun., 48 (1972) 743.

(6) L. A. Smets, Nature – New Biology 239 (1972) 123.

(7) G. S. Johnson and I. Pastan, Nature – New Biology 236 (1972) 247.

(8) J. Otten, G. S. Johnson and I. Pastan, Biochem. Biophys. Res. Commun., 44 (1972) 1192.

(9) J. Otten, G. S. Johnson and I. Pastan, J. Biol. Chem., 247 (1972) 7082.

(10) G. S. Johnson and I. Pastan, J. Nat. Cancer Inst., 47 (1972) 1357.

(11) G. S. Johnson, I. Pastan, C. V. Peery, J. Otten and M. Willingham, in: Prostaglandins in Cellular Biology, eds. P. Ramwell and B. Pharris (Plenum Press, N. Y., 1972) p. 195.

(12) J. R. Sheppard, Proc. Nat. Acad. Sci., U.S.A., 68 (1972) 1316.

(13) D. Paul, Nature – New Biology, 240 (1972) 179.

(14) A. Hsie and T. T. Puck, Proc. Nat. Acad. Sci., U.S.A., 68 (1972) 358.

(15) J. F. Goggins, G. S. Johnson and I. Pastan, J. Biol. Chem., 247 (1972) 5759.

CYCLIC AMP METABOLISM IN NORMAL AND TRANSFORMED FIBROBLASTS

I. PASTAN, M. WILLINGHAM, R. CARCHMAN AND W. B. ANDERSON
Laboratory of Molecular Biology
National Institutes of Health, National Cancer Institute

Abstract: The level of cyclic AMP correlates with the doubling time of growing cultured fibroblasts. Cyclic AMP levels rise at confluency in contact inhibited cells but not transformed cells. Serum, insulin and trypsin which stimulate growth lower cyclic AMP levels. Chick embryo cells recently transformed by Rous Sarcoma Virus have lower cyclic AMP levels than untransformed cells. This fall is accompanied by a fall in adenylate cyclase activity. The virus appears to stimulate the accumulation of a factor that changes the kinetic properties of adenylate cyclase.

Cyclic AMP has an important role in regulating the behavior and activity of cultured embryonic fibroblasts. The actions of cyclic AMP are most evident when transformed cells containing low cyclic AMP levels are treated with cyclic AMP analogues or prostaglandin $E_1$1. (For review see Reference 1) This paper will review recent work in our laboratory on the control of cyclic AMP levels in normal and transformed cells.

Embryonic fibroblasts and L-cells, like many other animal cells, contain an adenylate cyclase intimately associated with the plasma membrane. The enzyme is not activated by most polypeptide hormones but is activated by prostaglandin E_1 as well as some other prostaglandins (2).

47

Cyclic AMP is degraded by cyclic AMP phosphodiesterase.
On the basis of a kinetic analysis, chick embryo cells
appear to contain at least two different forms of the enzyme. One form with a low Km and specific for cyclic AMP
is associated with the plasma membrane. Another activity
with a higher Km for cAMP and able to hydrolyze cGMP is
present in the soluble fraction of the cell (3).

In a study of cyclic AMP levels in logarithmically
growing cells, Otten et al. (4) found that there was a
striking correlation between cyclic AMP levels and the
doubling time of cells. Cells with rapid growth had low
cyclic AMP levels and cells with slow growth high levels.
Of particular interest was the observation that cyclic AMP
levels were elevated in non-growing contact inhibited 3T3
cells, but not in confluent transformed cells in which
growth was continuing. This finding that cyclic AMP levels
rise in confluent untransformed cells has been extended to
a variety of cell lines including mouse 3T3-42 cells, (5)
normal rat kidney cells (NRK), (6), human diploid cells
(Wi38 and MA 308) (6, 7) and chick embryo fibroblasts (CEF)
(6). In chick embryo cells the rise in cyclic AMP levels
is accompanied by a rise in adenylate cyclase activity (8).

The density achieved by contact-inhibited cells is
regulated by the pH at which these cells are grown (9).
D'Armiento et al. (7) have measured the levels of cyclic
AMP in Wi38 cells grown at pH 6.6 or pH 7.7. The pH was
regulated by the addition of organic buffers to the growth
medium as described by Eagle and coworkers (9). At pH 6.6
where the saturation density was markedly lowered, the
cells accumulated very high levels of cyclic AMP (Fig. 1).
On the other hand, in confluent cells grown at pH 7.7, the
levels of cyclic AMP were not as strikingly elevated, but
were still much higher than the levels in logarithmically
growing cells.

The effect of a variety of factors that stimulate
growth have also been examined. These include serum, insulin and trypsin. Treatment of cultured cells with any of
these produces a rapid fall in cyclic AMP levels (5). An
example of the effect of serum on cyclic AMP levels is
shown in Fig. 2. Administration of serum to confluent
serum-starved 3T3 cells results in a rapid fall in

cyclic AMP levels followed by a wave of DNA synthesis some 20-25 hours later. The mechanism by which serum lowers cyclic AMP levels in CEF is under study.

In order to investigate the mechanism accounting for the low cyclic AMP levels in transformed cells, a variety of studies have been done on virally transformed mouse cells. In general these studies have been inconclusive (For review see Reference 10) One possible reason for these inconclusive results may be that the cells were carried in culture for many generations after transformation before they were studied. In order to circumvent this difficulty, we have begun to work with CEF which can be rapidly transformed by Rous Sarcoma Virus.

TABLE 1

Cyclic AMP content of chick embryo cells in culture

Cells	Growth Temperature	
	40.5°	36°
	(pmoles cAMP per mg nucleic acid)	
CEF	207 + 13	214 + 22
CEF-RSV-BH	39 + 3	34 + 3
CEF-RSV-BHTa	197 + 15	< 20

Table 1. From Reference 11, cells were grown at 40.5° and half the plates were shifted to 36° 12 hours before cyclic AMP was extracted. Cyclic AMP was extracted and assayed as previously described (4). The values shown are the mean + S. E. of mean.

CEF recently transformed by the Bryan High Titer strain of Rous Sarcoma Virus (RSV-BH) have much lower cyclic AMP levels than untransformed cells (Table 1). This fall in cyclic AMP levels is accompanied by a decrease in activity due to a marked change in the kinetic properties of adenylate cyclase (10). In general,

transformation results in an increase in the Km[ATP] from
0.2 mM in normal cells to 1.0 mM in transformed cells.
However, this isnnot the only change; there is also a
marked change in the Mg^{++} concentration dependence. The
adenylate cyclase of normal cells is usually saturated at
20 mM Mg^{++}, whereas that of RSV-BH CEF is saturated at
5 mM Mg^{++}.

Transformation also affects cyclic AMP phosphodiesterase activity. There is a significant increase in total
cAMP phosphodiesterase activity and in the ratio of low Km
to high Km enzyme on a Vmax basis, when the RSV transformed
cells are compared with normal cells.

We have also studied cAMP metabolism in a mutant
RSV in which the transformation function is temperature
sensitive (RSV-BH-Ta). Bader has found that cells
infected with RSV-BH-Ta and grown at 41°C appeared normal,
but only a few minutes after the cells were shifted to
36°C they began to morphologically transform (12).
Accompanying the transformation is a fall in cyclic AMP
levels (11). This fall in cyclic AMP levels is accompanied
by a change in the adenylate cyclase. The enzyme changes
from a form with relatively normal kinetic properties to
one with the properties of the transformed cells (10).

These findings suggest that the wild type virus produces a product that decreases adenylate cyclase activity.
Presumably in the mutant virus thevviral product is
temperature sensitive so that it is inactive at 41° but
capable of decreasing adenylate cyclase activity when the
cells are grown at 37°C. The nature of this putative
"transformation factor" is under study.

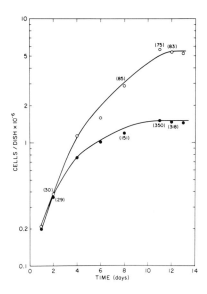

Fig. 1. Figure taken from Reference 7. Cyclic AMP levels in cells grown at pH 6.6 (O) or pH 7.7 (O). Media changed daily. The cyclic AMP levels in pmoles/mg nucleic acid are shown in parentheses.

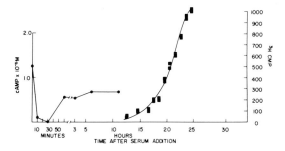

Fig. 2. Fall in cyclic AMP levels following serum addition. Taken from Reference 5.

51

REFERENCES

(1) G. S. Johnson - this volume.

(2) C. V. Peery, G. S. Johnson and I. Pastan, J. Biol. Chem., 246 (1971) 5785.

(3) T. R. Russell - in preparation.

(4) J. Otten, G. Johnson and I. Pastan, Biochem. Biophys. Res. Commun. 44 (1971) 1192.

(5) J. Otten, G. Johnson and I. Pastan, J. Biol. Chem., 247 (1972) 7082.

(6) R. Carchman - in preparation.

(7) D'Armiento, M., G. S. Johnson and I. Pastan, Nature, in press.

(8) W. B. Anderson - personal communication.

(9) C. Ceccarini and H. Eagle, Nature - New Biology 233 (1971) 271.

(10) W. Anderson, G. Johnson and I. Pastan, Proc. Nat. Acad. Sci. USA, in press, 1973.

(11) J. Otten, J. Bader, G. S. Johnson and I. Pastan, J. Biol. Chem., 247 (1972) 1632.

(12) J. P. Bader, Virology, 10 (1972) 267.

DISCUSSION

S. Assaf, University of Miami: I have not heard you describe any of the properties of the myosin-like protein which you have purified to homogeneity. Did you characterize it?

G.S. Johnson, National Institutes of Health: No, we have not characterized it.

S. Assaf: Did you study the effect of cyclic AMP-mediated phosphorylation on this protein?

G.S. Johnson: We have no data on the phosphorylation of myocin, but we are actively pursuing this possibility.

J.R. Sheppard, University of Colorado: What is the doubling time of the 3T3 cell in your hands?

I. Pastan, National Institutes of Health: Usually, it is somewhat less than 24 hours.

J.R. Sheppard: You have the density at day 4 which is about $\frac{1}{2}$ of the confluent density, and the next point that you take is at 8 days. Confluency should have occurred around 5. This is the important point where cyclic AMP should have been determined. Please, let me speculate what might be happening: if mucopolysaccharide is being produced by the 3T3 cell after confluency, possibly as the cell sits at confluency, the accumulation of the polysaccharide at the exterior of the cell then might interfere with, or inhibit transfer of nutrients which might lead to an increase of the cyclic AMP level.

I. Pastan: I'm going to show another slide to see
if it will help. At the time we did these experiments,
as you probably know, it was very difficult to measure
cyclic AMP levels, and we never know quite how to time
the experiment. But what I show is one typical experiment.
This is just the only other experiment I brought with me
in which we've measured cyclic AMP levels during growth.
It can be seen, on day 2 that the levels are low. At day
5 or 6, they are elevated. Perhaps this cell line is still
growing, slowing its growth with a level of 85. I agree
that we don't have perfect kinetics. I think that the weight
of the evidence, since cyclic AMP levels do rise at confluency
in so many cell lines, and since cyclic AMP levels correlate
with growth rates, favors the idea that it does mediate
contact inhibition of growth.

G. Cherayil, Milwaukee: I would like to direct this
question to Dr. Johnson. Would you please explain this
sentence in the abstract. It states that the "altered glycolipid
content of transformed cells is not changed". Was this
just total glycolipids that were measured?

G.S. Johnson: Transformed cell have different ganglioside content from that of normal cells. In collaboration
with Dr. Roscoe Brady, we found that dibutyryl cyclic
AMP didn't change the ganglioside pattern of L29 or 3T3-
Py11 cells.

P. Brown, Brown University: I think we all appreciate
your mention of the problems involved in assaying for
cyclic AMP. Have you ever used high-pressure liquid
chromatography to assay for cyclic AMP, or do you know
people who have, and what are the differences in assaying
results?

I. Pastan: I've never used high-pressure liquid chromatography. I believe Dr. Krishna, at NIH, is beginning.

G. Krishna, National Institutes of Health: We have used high-pressure liquid chromatography but it is in preliminary stages. I think I'd like to make a general comment regarding the measurements of cyclic AMP. All the assays that are being used with one exception, that of Dr. Ben Weiss, are purely biological assays even though they are called radioimmunoassay or the Gilman assay. They are what we are really measuring, the composition. For example, the immunoassay. I'm not sure Steiner had mentioned it, and I'm not sure people realize it, that other compounds are very similar to cyclic AMP. For example, 2' cyclic AMP can be present and would assay even though it is present in 1/100 the amount of cyclic AMP at 100 times higher fold concentration. We should all do these assays, as Dr. Pastan has mentioned, with another chemical assay, such as you said, high-pressure liquid chromatography may be the ideal. But again, the sensitive assay is not as good as the immunoassay or the Gilman assay. The assay should be carried out with purification on high-pressure liquid chromatography followed by the Gilman or Steiner assay.

I. Pastan: I want to indicate, if I may, that when you do the radioimmunoassay you make derivative at the 2' position, you couple that derivative to a protein and you make antibodies against this derivative. So really, the assay is better for the derivative than for the cyclic AMP and if in cells there are other molecules resembling cyclic AMP, a lot of us are going to be in trouble.

P. Brown: I have another question for Dr. Johnson. You mentioned using 8-bromo-cyclic GMP, and dibutyryl cyclic GMP. Did you ever use the plain cyclic GMP?

G.S. Johnson: Cyclic GMP also has no affect.

W.Y. Cheung, St. Jude's Children's Research Hospital: I have a question that I would like to direct to Dr. Pastan. I'm sure all of us are very much impressed by your elegant

work and you and your colleagues have also done very
nice work earlier in the E. coli system. This is the question
I would like to direct to you. In your early work on E.
coli, you found that cyclic AMP induces a variety of protein
synthetic systems. You proposed that the mechanism of
action was at the level of transcription, probably at the
promoter area of the operon region. In the cultured cells
that you just described you found that cyclic AMP inhibited
DNA synthesis. In you last comment before closing,
you mentioned some effects of cyclic AMP on cultured fibroblasts. I was wondering whether you would like to
relate the two systems that you have been working with
in the past few years. Do you think that the mode of action
of cyclic AMP, which is at the level of transcription in
the E. coli system, might also apply to the tissue cultures
that you just described?

I. Pastan: Well, when we began to work with cultured
cells, we thought that all of the techniques that we developed
and the knowledge that we developed studying E. coli
would enable us to study transcriptional control in animal
cells, but what we observed were rapid changes that
were not inhibited by inhibitors of either RNA or protein
synthesis. All the changes I've discussed today, except
with the possible exception of the induction of mucopolysaccharide synthesis, and some other data I haven't mentioned
by Dr. d'Armiento on the induction of phosphordiesterase
synthesis, occur very rapidly. And I'm reminded of the
story about Willie Sutton, a famous bank robber, when
asked why he robbed banks, said, "Well, that's where
the money is".

G. Krishna: I want to ask Dr. Pastan what he thinks
of the inhibitor which inhibits the cyclase and I wonder
if he has measured lactic acid or lactate in the medium,
since we have shown that lactate is one of the most important
inhibitors of cyclase under certain conditions.

I. Pastan: We have not studied the action of lactate
on adenylate cyclase, but we should have.

THE MOLECULAR CORRELATION CONCEPT OF NEOPLASIA

AND THE CYCLIC AMP SYSTEM

GEORGE WEBER

Department of Pharmacology, Indiana University
School of Medicine, Indianapolis, Indiana

Abstract: This paper discusses recent advances made by the
molecular correlation concept as a conceptual and experimental approach and describes the application to the
cAMP system.

In a model system of the spectrum of hepatomas
of different growth rates there was an ordered
pattern of gene expression that was manifested in the
imbalance of opposing and competing key enzymes and
overall metabolic sequences in the synthetic and degradative pathways of carbohydrate, pyrimidine, DNA and
cAMP metabolism. The metabolic imbalance was also expressed in a shift of the isozyme pattern. The metabolic imbalance was co-variant with hepatoma growth rate,
indicating the link between the proliferative and metabolic expression of the genes. The metabolic imbalance
confers selective biological advantages on the cancer
cells. The metabolic and enzymatic imbalance was specific to neoplasia and through the discriminating power
of the biochemical pattern it was demonstrated that no
similar pattern was present in the normal adult, fetal,
differentiating or regenerating liver. The conclusion
was reached that what is important about neoplasia is
ordered and what is not, is the random element and the
diversity.

INTRODUCTION

The objective of this presentation is to examine the question whether the approaches of the molecular correlation concept are applicable to the cyclic AMP system in normal and neoplastic cells. For this purpose first I will discuss the conceptual and experimental approaches of the molecular correlation concept of neoplasia and the main results and the conclusions that arose from this study. Then I will examine the applicability to the altered pattern of gene expression in neoplastic cells in the cyclic AMP system.

THE MOLECULAR CORRELATION CONCEPT: GENERAL AND SPECIAL

THEORIES

The general theory of the molecular correlation concept. This approach is concerned with elucidating the pattern and regulation of gene expression in physiological functions. It analyzes the link between the progressive expression and modulation of physiological functions and molecular events.

The special theory of the molecular correlation concept. This approach is concerned with the molecular correlates of malignancy. The special theory seeks to elucidate the pattern of regulation of gene expression in normal and neoplastic growth. It analyzes the link between the progressive degrees of malignant transformation and metabolic imbalance.

Conceptual and experimental approaches of the molecular correlation concept. In analyzing the pattern of gene expression and the possible linking between the extents in the expression of a function and the molecular events, there are five aspects that should be elucidated.

(1) There is need for delineation of the scope, biological role and degrees of expression of the physiological function studied. This step is of importance in the linking of the overall events in gene expression and the identification of co-variants of molecular events. (2) There is a need to identify the key quantitative discrim-

58

inants at the biochemical level that best correlate with
the various degrees of expression of a function. (3) In
analyzing the reprogramming of gene expression which is
entailed in the modulation of a function, it is necessary
to recognize the qualitative discriminants that characterize the varying extent of expression of a function. (4) It
should be possible to identify the integrated pattern of
gene expression that characterizes, as a syndrome, by an
array of quantitative and qualitative discriminants the
degrees in the expression of a function. (5) It is relevant to clarify the selective biological advantages that
the function, its regulation and the underlying molecular
events can provide for the biological system.

These five aspects that apply to the general theory
of the molecular correlation concept and the definition
of the term, discriminant, are discussed in detail elsewhere [1]. In this presentation our attention will focus
on the analysis of the molecular correlates of malignancy
that is the concern of the molecular correlation concept
of neoplasia [2-7].

Special Theory: The Molecular Correlation Concept of

Neoplasia

Malignancy is defined as "the ability of tumor cells
to grow progressively and kill their host" [8]. Table 1
summarizes the considerations relevant to the molecular
correlation concept of neoplasia.

MATERIALS AND METHODS

The preparation of homogenates, supernatant fluids,
slices, description of the hepatoma spectrum, biological
and biochemical properties and the different enzymatic and
metabolic assays are cited throughout this manuscript.
The reader is referred to the original publications and
the legends to Tables and Figures where further citations
are given.

TABLE 1

The special theory of the molecular correlation concept of neoplasia should identify the pattern in the following aspects of gene expression

1. DEGREES IN THE BIOLOGICAL BEHAVIOR OF CANCER CELLS:	the extent of expression of neoplastic transformation *
2. KEY QUANTITATIVE DISCRIMINANTS:	activities of opposing key enzymes and metabolic pathways
3. KEY QUALITATIVE DISCRIMINANTS:	shift in isozyme pattern; quantitative changes of several orders of magnitude; alterations opposite in direction to those of control tissues of similar growth rates
4. INTEGRATED PATTERN OF DISCRIMINANTS:	diagnostic pattern that specifically discriminates cancer cells from normal control tissues of similar growth rates (e.g., regenerating, differentiating or fetal tissues)
5. THE SELECTIVE BIOLOGICAL ADVANTAGE:	that the imbalance in control of gene expression for replication and for metabolic pattern confers to cancer cells

* Replicative function, growth rate.

60

SPECTRUM OF HEPATOMAS OF DIFFERENT MALIGNANCY: MODEL

SYSTEM FOR ELUCIDATION OF MOLECULAR BASIS OF NEOPLASTIC

TRANSFORMATION

In order to elucidate the link between neoplastic transformation and biochemical phenotype it was necessary to examine a biological model system where the degrees of neoplastic transformation can be studied in a graded, quantitative fashion. The spectrum of hepatomas of different growth rates [9] provided such a model system where the spheres of gene action, the indicators of reprogramming of gene expression and the degrees of metabolic imbalance can be correlated with the degrees in the expression of neoplastic transformation [2-7]. The progressive neoplastic departure from the biological behavior and the enzymatic and metabolic balance of the normal resting liver is reflected in the different degrees of altered gene expression in the different lines of liver tumors (Table 2).

Growth rate as a key factor. The malignancy of the transplanted hepatoma lines is measured by determining the growth rates of the neoplasms. Growth rate is an indicator of gene expression with which other indicators of gene expression in the biochemical phenotype are correlated. The significance of growth rate in neoplasia was given detailed attention elsewhere [1,7].

Tumor growth rate is measured by three independent methods which provide the ranking of the hepatomas (Table 3). Thus, it is an operational advantage to relate the biochemical events to the growth rate, because in this fashion all parameters that are compared are measured with precision.

The conceptual and experimental approaches of the molecular correlation concept of neoplasia were applied to the model system of hepatomas of different growth rates. The degrees in the expression of the imbalance in metabolism were compared with the degrees of expression of neoplastic transformation as measured in tumor growth rate. The results of the systematic, long-term investigation have been published elsewhere [1-7, 10-22], and now the main

TABLE 2

Spectrum of hepatomas of different malignancy: Model system for elucidation of molecular basis of neoplastic transformation

Spheres of Gene Action	Indicators of Reprogramming of Gene Expression	Degrees in Expression of Neoplastic Transformation Extent of Change from Normal		
		Slight	Intermediate	Extensive
BIOLOGICAL BEHAVIOR	Growth rate	Low	Medium	Rapid
MORPHOLOGY	Differentiation	Near normal	Medium	Poor
GENETIC APPARATUS	Chromosome number	Normal	Increased	High
	Chromosome karyotype	Normal	Altered	Deranged
ENERGY GENERATION	Respiration	Normal	Moderately low Normal or increased	Low
	Glycolysis	Low		High
REPLICATION AND FUNCTIONS	Imbalance in opposing pathways of synthesis and degradation	Moderate	Advanced	Pronounced
ISOZYME PATTERN	Isozyme shift	Moderate	Advanced	Pronounced

TABLE 3

Measuring growth rate in the hepatoma spectrum

BIOLOGICAL	size, weight, volume of tumors; time between transplantation
CYTOLOGICAL	mitotic counts
BIOCHEMICAL	ratio of TdR to DNA/TdR to CO_2

conclusions are presented in order to give an up-to-date picture and to provide a framework against which the behavior of the cyclic AMP system can be examined.

CARBOHYDRATE METABOLISM: PHENOTYPIC EVIDENCE FOR RE-

PROGRAMMING OF GENE EXPRESSION IN NEOPLASIA

The evidence for reprogramming of gene expression in carbohydrate metabolism in neoplastic liver is summarized in Table 4. The following alterations in carbohydrate metabolism occur in parallel with tumor growth rate. The key synthetic enzymes of gluconeogenesis decreased, whereas the key catabolic enzymes increased. As a consequence there emerged a metabolic imbalance where the ratios of activities of key glycolytic/key gluconeogenic enzymes markedly increased in parallel with hepatoma growth rate [19].

A pattern of isozyme shift was discovered for the key glycolytic enzymes that involved a decrease in the high K_m isozymes (glucokinase and liver-type pyruvate kinase) and an increase in the low K_m isozymes (hexokinase and the "muscle-type" pyruvate kinase). The relation of the metabolic imbalance and isozyme shift to growth rate was established in the hepatoma spectrum by recognizing that these alterations were co-variant with tumor growth rate [3,4,14]. These alterations are malignancy-linked characteristics and are indicators of the reprogramming of the

63

TABLE 4

Phenotypic evidence for reprogramming of gene expression in carbohydrate metabolism in neoplasia

1.	SYNTHETIC ENZYMES	Key gluconeogenic enzymes*	Decreased
2.	CATABOLIC ENZYMES	Key glycolytic enzymes**	Increased
3.	METABOLIC IMBALANCE	Ratios of key glycolytic/ key gluconeogenic enzymes	Increased
4.	ISOZYME SHIFT	High K_m isozymes+ Low K_m isozymes‡	Decreased Increased
5.	RELATION TO MALIGNANCY	Alterations are co-variant with growth rate	Malignancy linked imbalance
6.	BIOLOGICAL ROLE	(a) Imbalance in glycolytic/ gluconeogenic enzymes leads to increase in glycolysis	Confers selective advantages to cancer cells
		(b) Isozyme shift leads to decreased responsiveness to physiological controls	

* Glucose-6-phosphatase, fructose 1,6-diphosphatase, phosphoenolpyruvate carboxy-kinase, pyruvate carboxylase.

** Hexokinase, phosphofructokinase, pyruvate kinase.

+ Glucokinase, liver type pyruvate kinase.

‡ Hexokinase, muscle type pyruvate kinase.

genome. The progressive imbalance manifests the degrees
of gene expression in the biochemical phenotype which
parallels the progression in the extent of neoplastic
transformation.

An examination of the biological role of the altered
gene expression in carbohydrate metabolism indicates that
it confers a selective advantage to the cancer cells [4].
This conclusion is based on the fact that the imbalance
in the ratios of glycolytic/gluconeogenic enzymes leads to
a biochemical pattern that is favorable to glycolysis and
eliminates gluconeogenic recycling. In consequence, the
available glucose precursor can be used chiefly for glycolysis and observations carried out in this laboratory
first demonstrated that the glycolytic rate did increase
in parallel with the growth rate of the hepatomas [10, 11,
22]. It was also first recognized in this laboratory that
there was a pattern in the isozyme shift in neoplasia [3,
4]. The isozyme shift occurs in such a fashion that the
high K_m isozymes, that were subject to nutritional, hormonal and feedback controls, decreased, and were gradually
replaced by the low K_m isozymes that were not subject to
nutritional and hormonal regulation and much less targets
of allosteric regulation by physiological signals. In
consequence, the isozyme shift leads to a decreased responsiveness to physiological controls. This provides an
explanation at the molecular level for the tendency of
cancer cells to be less responsive to regulation [3,4].

Thus, these alterations confer selective advantages to
cancer cells in that they insure the predominance of glycolysis, eliminate the functioning of the opposing pathway,
gluconeogenesis, and result in a decreased susceptibility
to regulatory signals coming from other cells of the organ-
ism.

DNA METABOLISM: PHENOTYPIC EVIDENCE FOR REPROGRAMMING OF

GENE EXPRESSION IN NEOPLASIA

Since growth rate and replication are closely linked
with the operation and control of pyrimidine and DNA
metabolism, a systematic investigation was directed in my

TABLE 5

Comparison of activities of enzymes involved in anabolic
and catabolic pathways of pyrimidine and DNA metabolism

ENZYMES	LIVERS Normal fed*	Reg. 24 hr+	HEPATOMAS+ Rapidly growing Novikoff	3683F
ANABOLIC ENZYMES				
Ribonucleotide reductase	3		25,300	20,800
DNA polymerase	56	540		5,810
dTMP synthase	180	1,140	4,510	2,860
dTMP kinase	420	1,620	7,100	
TdR kinase	2,400	680	14,000	10,200
Uridine kinase	6,200	210		
dCMP deaminase	12,000	350	900	750
OMP pyrophosphorylase	20,000	380		
OMP decarboxylase	71,000			
CP synthase	94,000	96		
Aspartate transcarbamylase	123,000	127	480	796
Dihydro-orotase	246,000	108		418
Nucleosidediphosphate kinase	1,200,000			200
CATABOLIC ENZYMES				
Dihydrouracil dehydrogenase	26,000	78		9
Beta-ureido propionase	144,000	58		
Dihydrouracil hydrase	276,000	66		
TdR phosphorylase	234,000	106		31

Modified from Weber, et al. [19]. In order to achieve
a comparison all data were recalculated in μμmoles of substrate metabolized/mg protein/hr. In calculations the values of 0.2 g protein/g wet weight of tissue for homogenates and 0.08 g protein/g wet weight for supernatant fluids
were used.

* Values expressed as μμm/mg protein/hr.
+ Values expressed as % liver.

laboratories to discover the pattern and the relationship of these metabolic functions to the degrees of neoplastic transformation in the hepatoma spectrum. The details were published elsewhere [15-17,19,20] and the main results are summarized in the present work. Table 5 compares the activities of the synthetic and catabolic enzymes of pyrimidine and DNA metabolism, determined in my laboratories and in other centers [19]. A pattern was recognized in that the enzymes that exhibit the lowest activities in the normal liver are the ones that increased to the greatest extent in the most rapidly growing hepatomas (ribonucleotide reductase, DNA polymerase). The synthetic enzymes that have the highest activity in the resting liver exhibit the smallest extent of rise in the rapidly growing neoplasms (aspartate transcarbamylase, dihydro-orotase, nucleoside diphosphokinase). It is noteworthy that the enzymes of pyrimidine catabolism (dihydrouracil dehydrogenase, thymidine phosphorylase) have in general much higher activities than the rate-limiting enzymes of the synthetic pathways (the reductase in the de novo pathway; the DNA polymerase in the final common path of the de novo and salvage pathways). A comparison of absolute activities of "opposing enzymes" is done with great caution, since compartmentation, endogenous substrate levels, substrate transport and concentration as well as enzyme co-factors, pH and other metabolites might strongly influence the in vivo situation. Nevertheless, the conclusion drawn from this Table suggested to us that in the hepatoma spectrum one would predict an increase in the key synthetic enzyme activities that should parallel hepatoma growth rate and a decrease in the key catabolic enzyme activities that should negatively correlate with tumor growth rate. An analysis of the results obtained in this laboratory and data from other centers indicated that this prediction was correct [19].

The phenotypic evidence for the reprogramming of gene expression in nucleic acid metabolism is summarized in Table 6. The key enzymes of UMP, TTP and DNA synthesis increased in parallel with tumor growth rate; in contrast, the rate-limiting enzymes of UMP and TdR catabolism decreased in parallel with tumor growth rate. As a result, an imbalance arose between the synthetic and catabolic enzymes and between the overall pathways of synthesis and

TABLE 6

Phenotypic evidence for reprogramming of gene expression in DNA metabolism in neoplasia

1. SYNTHETIC ENZYMES	Key enzymes of UMP*, TTP** and DNA$^+$ synthesis	Increased
2. DEGRADATIVE ENZYMES	Key enzymes of UMP and TdR catabolism‡	Decreased
3. ENZYMATIC IMBALANCE	Ratios of synthetic/catabolic enzymes	Increased
4. METABOLIC IMBALANCE	Ratios of TdR to DNA/TdR to CO_2 pathways	Increased
5. RELATION TO MALIGNANCY	Alterations are co-variant with growth rate	Malignancy-linked imbalance
6. BIOLOGICAL ROLE	(a) Imbalance in anabolic/catabolic enzymes of UMP metabolism leads to increased de novo DNA synthesis (b) Imbalance in anabolic/catabolic enzymes of TdR metabolism leads to increased salvage pathway to DNA synthesis	Confers selective advantages to cancer cells

* Aspartate transcarbamylase, dihydro-orotase.
** Ribonucleotide reductase, dCMP deaminase, dTMP synthase, TdR kinase, dTMP kinase.
+ DNA polymerase
‡ Dihydrouracil dehydrogenase, dihydrothymine dehydrogenase.

degradation. This metabolic imbalance was especially clearly reflected in the close correlation between the ratios of the conversion of TdR to DNA/TdR to CO_2 and tumor growth rate [16]. The thymidine ratio showed the best correlation with growth rate among the biochemical factors examined to date and the ratios can be used to measure biochemically the growth rate in the hepatoma spectrum [19]. The enzyme that shows the greatest extent of rise and correlates the best with hepatoma growth rate was the ribonucleotide reductase shown by Elford [23]. Certain enzymatic and metabolic alterations in nucleic acid metabolism in the hepatoma spectrum were co-variant with growth rate. Thus, these parameters represent malignancy-linked phenotypic expressions of neoplasia.

The imbalance in the ratios of synthetic/catabolic enzymes of pyrimidine and DNA metabolism leads to a biochemical pattern that highly favors synthetic utilization of precursors and effectively eliminates recycling by the marked decrease and abolition of the key catabolic enzymes [16,19]. In consequence, the available precursors can be used chiefly for pyrimidine and DNA biosynthesis and the observations obtained by studying the ratio of disposition of thymidine for synthetic versus catabolic use is in good agreement with this prediction. Thus, in pyrimidine and DNA metabolism the reprogramming of gene expression confers selective advantages on the cancer cells by insuring the predominance of synthesis and by eliminating the functioning of the opposing catabolic pathways.

ORNITHINE METABOLISM: PHENOTYPIC EVIDENCE FOR REPRO-

GRAMMING OF GENE EXPRESSION IN NEOPLASIA

Ornithine occupies a central position in a metabolic crossroad. This amino acid is not contained in any of the proteins; therefore, as pointed out by Williams-Ashman, its function must lie elsewhere [24]. Ornithine may be channeled (a) into urea synthesis by ornithine carbamyl transferase activity; (b) or metabolized by ornithine decarboxylase, resulting in putrescine formation, or (c) metabolized by ornithine transaminase. Thus, ornithine is at the fountainhead of urea cycle and polyamine biosynthesis. Since the urea cycle competes with purine and pyrimidine biosynthesis for two important precursors (carbamyl phosphate, aspartate), it seemed that this competition might provide a target area for a metabolic imbalance in the hepatoma spectrum where a correlation with growth rate might be predicted [25,26]. Another important aspect of ornithine metabolism is the fact that it is the only known precursor for polyamine biosynthesis and in turn the study of this metabolic area could assist in throwing light on the role of polyamines in cell replication and neoplasia. A systematic study carried out in collaboration with H. Guy Williams-Ashman resulted in the discovery of an imbalance in ornithine metabolism that relates to hepatoma growth rate [25,26].

This investigation demonstrated that ornithine carbamyl transferase activity decreased in parallel with the increase in hepatoma growth rate [26]. In contrast, ornithine decarboxylase increased in most of the hepatomas and there was an indication for an increase in the levels of certain polyamines [25]. The ratio of ornithine decarboxylase/ornithine carbamyl transferase increased in parallel with hepatoma growth rate [25,26].

Current preliminary studies in my laboratories in collaboration with Dr. Nobuhiko Katunuma (Tokushima University, Japan) and Dr. Ikuko Tomino (Jikei University, Japan) suggest that ornithine transaminase activity decreased in parallel with hepatoma growth rate, exhibiting low activities in rapidly growing neoplasms (to be published).

The biological importance of the imbalance in ornithine metabolism can be perceived from these results and it is illustrated in Figure 1. Of the metabolic pathways of ornithine, only ornithine decarboxylase is retained and increased in liver tumors. Since there is a decrease in ornithine carbamyl transferase activity, a decrease should occur in the utilization of carbamyl phosphate and aspartate for urea synthesis and consequently these precursors could be preferentially spared for the synthesis of DNA and RNA. The results of Sweeney et al. showed that the first two enzymes of orotate synthesis (aspartate transcarbamylase, dihydro-orotase) increased in parallel with hepatoma growth rate [27], indicating that these precur-

70

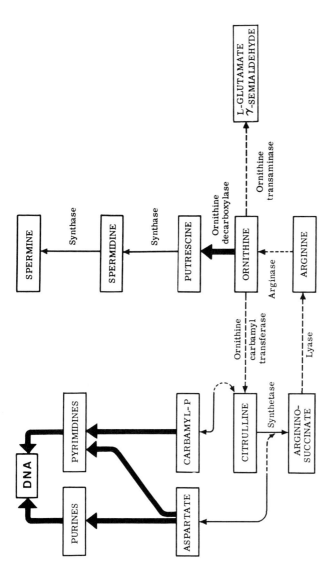

Fig. 1. Biological selective advantages that an imbalance in ornithine metabolism may confer to cancer cells. Modified from (20).

71

sors might indeed be preferentially utilized for nucleic acid biosynthesis. Thus, the metabolic imbalance in the ratios of ornithine decarboxylase/ornithine carbamyl transferase might confer a selective biological advantage on the cancer cells as this imbalance becomes progressively more pronounced with the increase in tumor growth rate. Thus, in the area of ornithine metabolism the phenotypic evidence indicates a reprogramming of gene expression that is linked with tumor growth rate and confers a biological advantage on neoplastic cells [25,26].

SPECIFICITY OF METABOLIC PHENOTYPE TO MALIGNANCY

In order to investigate the specificity of the alterations in gene expression to neoplasia it is necessary to examine the biochemical pattern in a series of control tissues that exhibit similar biological properties in terms of growth rate. For this reason, the rapidly growing hepatomas are selected because in these very malignant neoplasms we observe the extreme expression of the enzymatic and metabolic imbalance. The control tissues are provided by the rapidly growing regenerating liver in the adult rat, the near-term (19-day-old) differentiating embryonic liver and the developing liver of the 6-day-old rat. The various considerations governing the selection of these control tissues are outlined elsewhere [1-7].

In Table 7 the enzyme activities were calculated in μmoles of substrate metabolized per hr per gram wet weight of tissue and expressed as μmoles of substrate metabolized per hr per average cell. In order to allow a comparison the results are given in the Table in percentages, taking the values of the liver of the adult rat as 100%. For the absolute values of enzyme activities, reference is made to publications cited in this paper.

The operative terminology employed for discriminating the alterations in the various tissues and the term "discriminant" are defined elsewhere [1].

72

TABLE 7

Discriminating power of biochemical pattern:
Key differences between rapidly growing neoplastic, fetal,
newborn and regenerating liver

Markers of gene expression	Liver			
	Neoplastic (rapidly growing)	Newborn (6-day-old)	Fetal (17 days old)	Regenerating (24 hr)
TdR into DNA	3,900	1,224*	3,083	910*
TdR to CO_2	<0.1	68+	5	64+
TdR to DNA/ TdR to CO_2	11,500,000	1,788*	54,550*	1,450+
DNA/cell	250	87		100
TdR Phosphorylase	32		2.0+	126
Ur Phosphorylase	375		1.8+	106
DUDH	<10			78
TdR kinase/ DUDH	>1,000			<10
OCT	<1	33+	6.6+	83+
G-6Pase	<1	350+	12+	100+
FDPase	<1	175+	7.1+	100+
PEP CK	<1	160+		100+
PC	<1	275+		100+
HK	500	36	83+	100+
PFK	229	44	49+	100+
PK	499	15	11+	100+
G-6-PDH	751	50	26+	100+
6PGDH	48	18	26	100+
HK/G-6-Pase	8,800	57+	690+	100+
PFK/FDPase	6,463	86+	674+	100+
G-6-PDH/6PGDH	1,120	288*	100+	100+

*Quantitative discriminant
+Qualitative discriminant
Values are expressed as percent of normal adult liver.

Discriminating Power of Biochemical Pattern: Key Differ-

ences Between Rapidly Growing Neoplastic, Fetal, Newborn

and Regenerating Liver

Contrasting the enzymatic and metabolic imbalance in the rapidly growing hepatomas with the pattern found in the normal liver demonstrates the vastly different bio-chemical phenotype of the cancer cell. It is also possible to readily discriminate between the biochemical pattern of the hepatoma cells and that of the regenerating liver. An examination of Table 7 and critical evaluation of results in the literature indicates that the difference between the biochemical phenotype of neoplastic liver and embryonic liver can be readily discerned. Similarly, the phenotype of the developing newborn liver and that of the hepatoma can be clearly discriminated. It is important to note the discriminating power of the biochemical pattern since there have been suggestions that neoplasia is a disease of differentiation or an emergence of an embryonic biochemical pattern. While there might be some coincidental over-lappings in the biochemical pattern, it is more important that the critical examination demonstrates numerous key differences between the biochemical phenotype of the hepa-tomas and that of the differentiating or embryonic liver.

The conclusion drawn from these considerations is that there is a diagnostic pattern of quantitative and qualita-tive discriminants that can specifically distinguish cancer cells from normal control tissues of similar growth rates, such as the regenerating, differentiating or fetal tissues. Thus, the evidence indicates that the molecular pattern of the cancer cells is ordered, it is linked with the degree of malignancy and it is specific to neoplasia.

SUMMARY OF PHENOTYPIC EVIDENCE FOR REPROGRAMMING OF GENE

EXPRESSION IN CANCER CELLS

The experimental results allow us to draw the follow-ing conclusions with application of the approaches of the special theory of the molecular correlation concept (Table

TABLE 8

Phenotypic evidence for reprogramming of gene expression in cancer cells

1. METABOLIC IMBALANCE:	in activities of opposing key enzymes and metabolic pathways
2. SHIFT IN ISOZYME PATTERN:	decrease in high K_m and increase in low K_m isozymes
3. DECREASED RESPONSIVENESS TO REGULATION:	hormonal stimulation, feedback and allosteric controls
4. RELATION TO BIOLOGICAL BEHAVIOR (MALIGNANCY):	biochemical alterations are progressive and correlate with growth rate

8). A metabolic imbalance is revealed in the activities of opposing key enzymes and metabolic pathways of synthesis and catabolism in the areas of carbohydrate, pyrimidine, DNA and ornithine metabolism. There is a shift in isozyme pattern, revealing a decrease in the high K_m and an increase in the low K_m isozymes in carbohydrate metabolism. A decreased responsiveness to regulation is revealed in a decline in responsiveness to hormonal stimulation, feedback and allosteric controls. Thus, in the metabolic phenotype the reprogramming of gene expression is linked with the progressive increase in malignancy as revealed in the hepatoma spectrum of tumors of different growth rates.

The above outlined analysis of the results of the experimental and conceptual approaches achieved by the molecular correlation concept of neoplasia indicated an ordered and specific pattern of gene expression in the hepatoma spectrum. Now we will examine the applicability of this pattern of malignancy-linked metabolic imbalance to the cyclic AMP system in hepatomas.

APPLICATION OF THE MOLECULAR CORRELATION CONCEPT TO THE CYCLIC AMP SYSTEM IN HEPATOMAS

In order to test the applicability of the molecular correlation concept of neoplasia to the cAMP system, the following approaches were employed. If the reprogramming of gene expression is also manifested in the cAMP system and if it resembles that observed for carbohydrate, pyrimidine, DNA and ornithine metabolism, the solution of the following problems may provide an insight. (1) An imbalance in cAMP metabolism could emerge as a consequence of an alteration in the ratio of the activities of the synthetic enzyme (adenylate cyclase) and the catabolic enzyme (cAMP phosphodiesterase) that determine the steady state level of cAMP. (2) An isozyme shift would be revealed by studying the responsiveness to regulation and the kinetic behavior of the synthetic and catabolic enzymes. (3) The biological significance of an anticipated imbalance might be reflected in the effects of addition of cAMP to cells in tissue culture and in the assays of cAMP levels in neoplasms. (4) In order to elucidate a possible linking with malignancy, the spectrum of transplantable hepatomas of different growth rates should be used as a model system where alterations in gene expression may be studied in a graded, quantitative fashion.

It is recognized that the experimental validity of these approaches depends on the suitability of the biological system and the various methods directed to the resolution of these problems. A further difficulty arises from the need, as yet not completely answered, that all parts of the system, such as the AMP level, the cyclase, the phosphodiesterase, and their responsiveness and steady state levels be measured in the same sub-cellular compartment, in the cellular membrane. The present report will deal chiefly with the studies undertaken in my laboratories, in part in collaboration with members of this Department, and some of these investigations are in the process of publication in full detail elsewhere.

Effect of cAMP on Hepatomas in Tissue Culture

The effect of cAMP was investigated on cell lines of slow growing hepatoma 8999 and rapidly growing hepatoma 3924A. In order to carefully delineate the possible action of cAMP, great care was taken to employ suitable controls. The properties of the two tumors in vivo and in tissue culture will be described in detail elsewhere. The two lines exhibited markedly different growth rates in the rat where hepatomas 8999 and 3924A required 4 and 1 months, respectively, to reach about one inch in diameter. The growth rate in tissue culture for hepatomas 8999 and 3924A was measured by the doubling times which were 28 ± 3 and 14 ± 0.6 hrs, respectively. The results of this preliminary study (S. F. Queener and G. Weber) are summarized in Table 9. When added alone to the incubation medium, up to a concentration of 1 mM, cAMP and 5'-AMP had relatively little effect; DBcAMP and butyric acid caused 25 and 35% inhibition, respectively. However, in presence of theophylline cAMP exhibited a dose-dependent inhibitory action. DBcAMP was also inhibitory and at the higher concentration (1 mM) the hepatoma cells were killed. It is of interest that butyric acid also showed a dose-related progressive inhibitory action which was not very different from that of DBcAMP. 5'-AMP in presence of theophylline also caused a pronounced inhibition at 1 mM concentration. Theophylline alone had a minor effect of 25 and 20% inhibition, respectively, for hepatomas 8999 and 3924A.

These studies draw attention to the fact that theophylline is required for the expression of cAMP inhibitory action and that butyric acid may well play a role in the inhibitory effects ascribed to DBcAMP. This type of effect is usually ascribed to an inhibitory action of theophylline on the phosphodiesterase activity; however, in the concentration employed it would not inhibit completely the powerful action of phosphodiesterase. Great caution is required in the interpretation of such experiments, since current work in this laboratory suggests that theophylline may act as a competitive inhibitor of thymidine uptake and butyric acid can inhibit the enzymes involved in glucose utilization. The results of current investigations on the effect of butyric acid will now be described in some detail.

TABLE 9

Effect of N^6-O^2-dibutyryl-3'5': cyclic AMP and related compounds on in vitro population doubling times of two hepatoma lines of different growth rates

Compounds	Concentration (mM)	Hepatoma 8999 Slow-growing		Hepatoma 3924A Rapidly-growing	
Controls	0.00	100 ± 5	(5)	100 ± 5	(9)
cAMP	0.01	–		100	(1)
	0.10	–		100	(1)
	1.00	–		100	(1)
DBcAMP	1.00	69 ± 10	(3)	75	(2)
5'AMP	1.00	–		100	(1)
Butyric acid	1.00	–		65	(1)
Theophylline	1.00	75 ± 10	(3)	80 ± 5	(6)
+ cAMP	0.01	–		72	(1)
	0.10	–		50 ± 9	(3)
	0.30	–		47 ± 11	(3)
	1.00	–		32 ± 10	(3)
+ DBcAMP	0.01	55	(1)	85	(2)
	0.10	20	(1)	66 ± 6	(3)
	0.30	–		40 ± 13	(2)
	1.00	0*	(4)	0**	(5)
+ Butyric acid	0.01	–		94	(1)
	0.10	–		68	(2)
	0.30	–		74	(1)
	1.00	42 ± 4	(3)	18 ± 9	(5)
+ 5'AMP	1.00	53	(1)	61	(1)

*Cells are killed, with a half-life of 85 ± 4 hours.
**Cells are killed, with a half-life of 73 hours.
Growth rates are expressed as population doubling times obtained from the slope of the logarithmic portion of the growth curves. Relative growth rate is the ratio of control doubling time/experimental doubling time X 100. Cells used were hepatoma 8999, culture generation 8-17 and hepatoma 3924A, culture generation 100-120. Figures in parenthesis are the number of independent determinations.

The Effect of Butyric Acid on Enzymes of Carbohydrate

Metabolism

Previous work from this laboratory showed that free fatty acids selectively inhibited the key enzymes of glycolysis and of the direct oxidative pathway and certain enzymes of the Krebs cycle but did not affect key enzymes of gluconeogenesis [28,29]. These studies were carried out in normal liver and in hepatomas of different growth rates and the inhibitory effects of free fatty acids on glycolysis were also demonstrated. The selective inhibition of a similar group of enzymes by free fatty acids was also shown in a microbial system employing Arthrobacter crystallopoietes [30]. Both the mammalian and microbial studies were carried out with fatty acids of longer chain length; butyric acid was not included in the investigations.

In the present standard assay system butyric acid was added to 100,000 X g supernatant fluid prepared from homogenates of normal liver and hepatoma 3924A as described elsewhere [28,29]. On incubation at 37^0 both glucokinase and hexokinase exhibit a time-dependent decrease in activity. However, addition of butyric acid to the incubation mixture caused a dose-dependent, much more marked decline in the enzyme activities. The results were corrected for the decrease observed in absence of butyric acid and the data are presented in Figures 2 and 3.

The dose-dependent action of butyric acid on glucokinase and hexokinase was examined after a 60-min preincubation period (Fig. 2). For the hexokinase of liver and hepatoma 3924A, K_i = 0.7 and 0.3 mM, respectively, was observed. For glucokinase in liver and hepatoma 3924A, K_i = 0.1 and 0.03 mM, respectively, was observed. These results indicate that the high K_m regulatory enzyme, glucokinase, is 7 to 10 times more sensitive to butyric acid than the low K_m isozyme, hexokinase.

A time-sequence study was carried out in presence of the concentration that was established to yield an apparent K_i in 60 min (Figure 3). The results confirm the dose-dependent inhibitory studies shown in Figure 2, also demonstrating that a 50% decrease in enzyme activities was

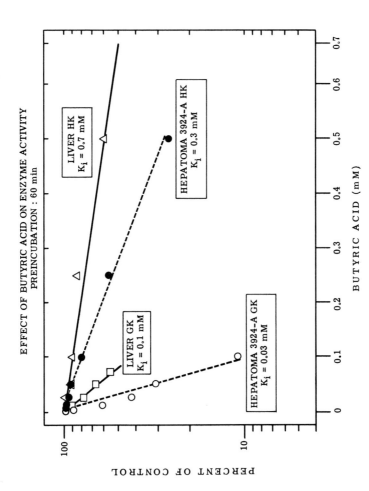

Fig. 2. Dose response studies. Effect of butyric acid on glucokinase and hexokinase activities of liver and hepatoma 3924A. A preincubation time of 60 min at 37° C was used.

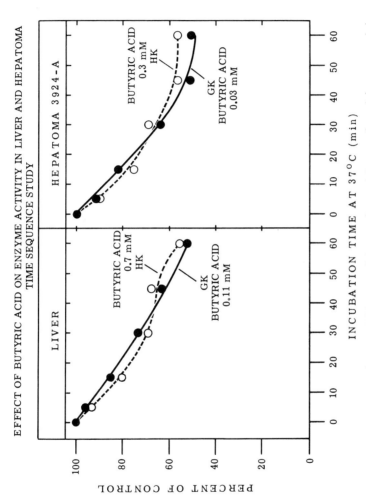

Fig. 3. Time sequence studies. Effect of butyric acid on glucokinase and hexokinase activities of liver and hepatoma 3924A. The concentrations of the butyric acid chosen were those of the apparent K_i indicated in Figure 2.

reached in 60 min. The decrease in enzyme activities was a progressive one.

These investigations indicate that the glucose phosphorylating enzymes in both normal liver and the rapidly growing hepatoma can be inhibited in a time- and dose-dependent fashion by butyric acid. These experiments caution that the liberation of butyric acid that should occur after addition of DBcAMP to tissue culture may cause a multiplicity of metabolic effects that may not be attributed to cAMP, but have their own action that may well be independent from DBcAMP.

Nevertheless, cAMP (in presence of theophylline) is able to exert an inhibitory effect on hepatoma cells in a dose-dependent fashion (Table 7). It is not necessary to emphasize the limited nature of the interpretative power of this type of results obtained in tissue culture regarding the potential homeostatic role or biological effectiveness of any compound examined. The results, however, are of interest and require further investigation.

Behavior of Adenylate Cyclase in Hepatomas of Different

Growth Rates

Investigations in our laboratories demonstrated that the basal levels of adenylate cyclase in hepatomas of different growth rates were unaltered from activities observed in control normal rat livers. Addition of sodium fluoride to the enzyme assay system resulted in an 8- to 10-fold increase in cyclase activity in all examined normal and neoplastic livers. However, the studies determining the sensitivity to glucagon stimulation showed a different pattern. Addition of glucagon to the assay system caused an increase to 236 to 343% in the normal livers and in the slow growing hepatomas. The extent of stimulation decreased in the medium growth rate tumors and there was no significant glucagon stimulation in the more rapidly growing hepatomas [31]. Thus, the responsiveness to glucagon stimulation declined with the increase in hepatoma growth rate (Table 10).

TABLE 10

Behavior of adenyl cyclase activity in normal and regenerating liver and in hepatomas of different growth rates

Tissues	No. experi-ments	Adenyl cyclase activity				
		$\mu mole/g/hr$*	NaF stimulated		Glucagon stimulated	
			$\mu mole/g/hr$*	% control	$\mu mole/g/hr$*	% control
Liver						
Normal (Holtzman)	14	0.14±0.02	1.30±0.12**	929	0.40±0.03**	286
Normal (Buffalo)	14	0.12±0.02	0.98±0.03**	815	0.41±0.03**	342
Normal (ACI/N)	10	0.07±0.01	0.74±0.02**	1050	0.24±0.02**	343
Sham-operated (Holtzman)	8	0.13±0.01	1.32±0.07**	1015	0.43±0.05**	307
Regenerating (Holtzman)	8	0.14±0.01	1.15±0.03**	821	0.33±0.01**	236
Hepatomas						
9618B(slow)+	4	0.07±0.01	0.82±0.10**	1171	0.31±0.08**	442
7787(slow)	4	0.07±0.03	0.90±0.18**	1285	0.22±0.08**	310
5123-tc(medium)	4	0.09±0.02	0.94±0.09**	1044	0.18±0.02**	200
7288C(medium)	6	0.08±0.01	0.39±0.06**	488	0.11±0.02	138
3924A(rapid)	10	0.12±0.01	0.72±0.09**	600	0.12±0.01	100
9618A2(rapid)	8	0.08±0.02	0.80±0.09**	1000	0.06±0.02	75

*Mean ± S.E. **Significantly different from control without stimulation ($p < 0.05$).
+Growth rate (9). (From: Allen, Munshower, Morris and Weber, Cancer Res. 31, 557-560, 1971.) Reaction mixture contained MgCl, 2.5 μmole; ATP-8-14C, 0.5 μmole, 0.5 μCi; theophylline, 5.0 μmole; trisodium 2-PEP, 3.0 μmole; PK, 1.5 units; tissue homogenate, 7.5 mg wet wt and appropriate drugs in Tris buffer, 25 mM, pH 7.4. The concentration of NaF was 10^{-2} M and glucagon was 10^{-6} M. Incubation period was 15 min at 37°. cAMP was isolated by method of Krishna et al. (32). The reaction was linear with time for at least 15 min under all conditions and was proportional to the amount of tissue within the range of amounts used.

The behavior of adenylate cyclase in regenerating liver was similar to that in the control normal tissues in every respect. Therefore, the decreased responsiveness to glucagon stimulation in the rapidly growing tumors is characteristic of the neoplastic transformation and it is not due to rapid growth rate alone, since the regenerating liver which has the same growth rate as the rapidly growing tumors shows no loss of glucagon responsiveness [31]. The loss of glucagon responsiveness is in line with the decreased regulatory responsiveness of various systems in the more rapidly growing hepatomas. The interpretation at the molecular level requires caution, since it might be an indication of an alteration in isozyme balance, or of the loss of a hormone receptor site or of the existence of two or more separate adenylate cyclase systems in the liver. Furthermore, it should be pointed out that the enzyme was assayed in the total homogenate and overall behavior of the total cyclase activity may mask the more specific and relevant alterations that might occur in the cell membrane. The importance of compartmentation is highly relevant here and the results of Rethy [33] and Tomasi [34] at this Conference indicate that the adenylate cyclase activity in the membrane of the rapidly growing hepatomas was decreased. These observations further emphasize the need to investigate the whole cyclase system in the different compartments of normal and neoplastic cells. The decrease in glucagon responsiveness of adenylate cyclase that parallels the increase in tumor growth rate is in line with what one would expect from the point of view of the molecular correlation concept of neoplasia.

The Behavior of cAMP Phosphodiesterase Activity in Hepato-

mas of Different Growth Rates

The phosphodiesterase activity was determined in 100,000 X $\underline{g}$ supernatant fluid at 1 mM cAMP (high K_m enzyme) and at 1 μM cAMP (low K_m enzyme) [35]. The results of kinetic studies and of enzyme assays at two cAMP concentrations suggest, but do not prove rigorously, that there are present in normal liver and in slow and rapidly growing hepatomas two phosphodiesterases, one with a low apparent K_m = 2 to 3 μM and another with an apparent K_m = 100 to 500 μM for cAMP (Fig. 4).

84

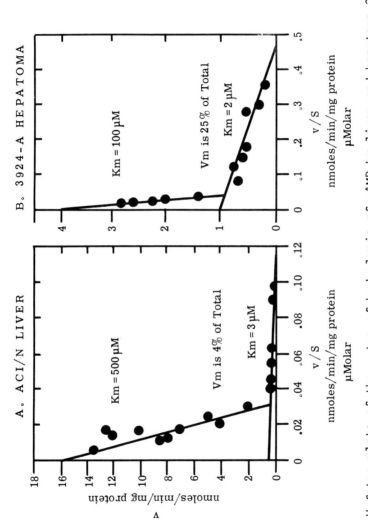

Fig. 4. Hofstee plots of the rates of hydrolysis of cAMP by liver and hepatoma 3924A supernatant fluid. The slope is the negative value for the apparent K_m and the intercept on the ordinate is the value for the apparent V_{max}. From [35].

TABLE 11

Cyclic AMP phosphodiesterase : Isozyme shift in hepatomas

Tissues	cAMP phosphodiesterase activity (%)	
	at 1 mM cAMP (High K_m enzyme)	at 1 µM cAMP (Low K_m enzyme)
Normal liver	100	100
Newborn liver (5 day)	38*	28*
Regenerating liver (24 hr)	154*	114
Hepatoma 47-C (slow)	58*	185*
Hepatoma 3924A (rapid)	13*	265*

* Significantly different from respective control tissue.

Activity of normal liver of adult Buffalo rat: at 1 mM cAMP = 40.6 ± 4.1; at 1 µM cAMP = 0.21 ± 0.02 µmoles/hr/g. From [35].

The high K_m phosphodiesterase activity was decreased in the slowly growing hepatoma 47-C and in the rapidly growing hepatoma 3924A to 58 and 13%, respectively, of the values of normal livers. In contrast, the low K_m phosphodiesterase activity in the slow and rapidly growing hepatomas increased to 185 and 265%, respectively (Table 11).

This alteration in the isozyme pattern of cAMP phosphodiesterase is specific to the neoplastic process, inasmuch as no similar isozyme shift was observed in the rapidly growing differentiating or regenerating liver [35].

The behavior of the cAMP phosphodiesterase isozyme is in line with the isozyme shift pattern in the high and low K_m glucokinase-hexokinase and pyruvate kinase systems. Thus, the observation for the phosphodiesterase isozyme shift supports the predictions of the molecular correlation concept that the neoplastic transformation entails a progressive emergence of a reprogramming of gene expression that appears to be linked with tumor growth rate.

The results of Rethy [33] and Tomasi [34] indicate that in the rapidly growing hepatoma the phosphodiesterase activity in the membrane is markedly increased. This observation further underlines the need for assaying the whole cAMP system in the membrane of normal and neoplastic cells for a more meaningful comparison and interpretation.

cAMP metabolism: phenotypic evidence for reprogramming of gene expression in neoplasia. The following considerations are relevant. If cAMP is a physiological inhibitor of growth or replicatory processes, its level should be decreased either as an overall concentration or at least at the relevant cellular compartment which may be the cell membrane, but it could be other locations such as for instance, the nucleolar membrane. Assays carried out in freeze clamp studies in collaboration with Drs. J. Ashmore and D. O. Allen in this Department in 3 separate experiments involving 36 samples of the rapidly growing hepatoma 3924A indicated that the total concentration of cAMP was the same as that observed in the liver of control normal rats (J. Ashmore, D. O. Allen and G. Weber, unpublished observations). However, the cAMP level may well be different in some critical area such as in the cell membrane.

If in spite of the preliminary evidence that there is no change in the overall concentration of cAMP, in considering the inhibitory action of cAMP in tissue culture (Table 9) one would be led to postulate an imbalance of the cyclase/phosphodiesterase enzyme system which might be reflected in the cell membrane. A contrasting of the absolute activities of adenylate cyclase and phosphodiesterase in the liver draws attention to the fact that at optimum substrate concentration these two opposing enzymes are very unequally poised. The activity of the phosphodiesterase is several orders of magnitude higher than that of the cyclase. However, the cyclase level can be increased by glucagon or epinephrine stimulation. Nevertheless, physiological inhibitors for phosphodiesterase activity would play a role in the balance if such modulators exist.

The fact that the adenylate cyclase activity in the rapidly growing hepatomas was no longer responsive to glucagon stimulation indicated that these tumors are not able to increase their potential of producing cAMP. Moreover, the fact that in the rapidly growing tumor, the phosphodiesterase with higher substrate affinity is the predominant isozyme which shows an increased activity, is an indication for an altered balance in the cyclase/phosphodiesterase system that could lead to a lowered cAMP generating capacity.

Studies in the membrane of rapidly growing hepatomas demonstrated that the membrane-bound adenylate cyclase decreased, whereas the phosphodiesterase activity increased [33,34]. This provides evidence for the operation of an imbalance in the cAMP generating and degradative systems in the membrane compartment. These observations are in line with the imbalance expected on the basis of the molecular correlation concept.

The evidence for the reprogramming of gene expression in neoplasia as it is manifested in the cAMP system is summarized in Table 12. The evidence is suggestive that the pattern of alterations is similar to that discovered for carbohydrate, pyrimidine, DNA and ornithine metabolism. Thus, the enzyme involved in the synthesis of cAMP is unaltered in the total homogenate, but is decreased in the cell membrane of the rapidly growing hepatomas. In contrast, the activity of the catabolic enzyme, phosphodiesterase, is increased in the cell membrane. A decrease in susceptibility to regulatory influence and the operation of an isozyme shift were recognized in the decrease in glucagon sensitivity for the cyclase and in the increased low K_m phosphodiesterase activity in the rapidly growing hepatomas. It appears that the imbalance in the cAMP system relates to the malignancy of the hepatomas.

The present results, interesting as they are, can only be taken as an indication that the alterations in the cAMP system are similar to those in other areas of imbalance in intermediary metabolism and in the opposing enzyme system as described by the molecular correlation concept of neoplasia. However, a great deal remains to be done before much firmer conclusions may be drawn, especially regarding

TABLE 12

Phenotypic evidence for reprogramming of gene expression in cAMP metabolism in hepatomas

1. cAMP LEVEL	Overall concentration, subcellular compartmentation, turnover	Not certain
2. SYNTHETIC ENZYME	Adenylate cyclase	
	Total cell activity	Unchanged
	-Sensitivity to NaF stimulation	Unchanged
	-Sensitivity to glucagon stimulation	Decreased with increase in growth rate
	Activity in membrane	Decreased
3. CATABOLIC ENZYME	cAMP phosphodiesterase	
	-Total soluble activity	Decreased
	-Activity in membrane	Increased
4. ISOZYME SHIFT	Glucagon responsive cyclase	Decrease in hormone sensitivity
5. ENZYMATIC IMBALANCE	Phosphodiesterase	
	-High K_m isozyme	Decreased
	-Low K_m isozyme	Increased
	Hormone responsive cyclase	Decreased
	Low K_m phosphodiesterase Activity in membrane	Increased
	-Adenyl cyclase	Decreased
	-Phosphodiesterase	Increased
	-Phosphodiesterase/cyclase ratio	Increased
6. BIOLOGICAL ROLE	Imbalance in membrane phosphodiesterase/cyclase ratio Isozyme shifts for phosphodiesterase and cyclase	Might confer selective advantages

89

the possible role of the cAMP system in the core of neoplastic transformation.

CONCLUSIONS

The objective of this paper was to discuss recent advances made by the molecular correlation concept as an experimental and conceptual tool and to describe the application of this approach to the cAMP system. The results provide evidence for the following conclusions.

(1) Ordered pattern of gene expression: metabolic imbalance. In a model system of the spectrum of hepatomas of
different growth rates, there is an ordered pattern of gene
expression that is manifested in the imbalance of opposing
and competing key enzymes and of overall metabolic sequences in the synthetic and degradative pathways.

(2) Isozyme shift. The metabolic imbalance is also expressed in the shift of isozyme pattern in which there
emerges a predominance of the low K_m enzymes (cAMP phosphodiesterase, hexokinase, muscle-type pyruvate kinase). Con-
currently, with the decrease or disappearance of the high
K_m enzymes that are subject to nutritional, hormonal, and
feedback regulation, the emergence of a series of low K_m
isozymes resulted in the decreased regulatory response exhibited by cancer cells. The decreased sensitivity to hormonal control is also manifested in the behavior of adenylate cyclase which gradually loses its responsiveness to
glucagon stimulation with the increase in hepatoma growth
rate. The behavior of the synthetic and degradative enzymes that play a key role in cyclic AMP homeostasis in the
hepatoma cell membrane is in line with the pattern anticipated by the approaches of the molecular correlation concept.

(3) Co-variance of metabolic imbalance with tumor
growth rate. The enzymatic and metabolic imbalance is co-
variant with hepatoma growth rate, indicating a link in the
metabolic and proliferative expression of the genes. Since
tumor growth rate is an important determinant of the susceptibility of human tumors to chemotherapy, the discovered
growth rate-linked metabolic imbalance should provide targets for the strategy of anti-cancer chemotherapy.

(4) Selective biological advantages of the imbalance
in gene expression. The metabolic imbalance confers a

selective biological advantage on the cancer cells by the progressive predominance of the synthetic pathway over the decrease in the degradative one in pyrimidine and nucleic acid metabolism. Through a gradually emerging imbalance in ornithine metabolism, the competition of the urea cycle for aspartate and carbamyl phosphate might be gradually switched off, permitting an increase in channeling of these precursors to biosynthesis of nucleic acids and polyamines. The imbalance in the cAMP system at the cell membrane level might favor neoplastic proliferation.

(5) Specificity of metabolic imbalance to neoplasia. The metabolic and enzymatic imbalance discovered in the hepatoma spectrum is specific to neoplasia, since no similar pattern is present in the fetal, differentiating, regenerating or normal liver.

(6) Discriminating power of the biochemical pattern. The enzymatic and metabolic imbalance provides quantitative and qualitative discriminants that allow the recognition of the differences at the molecular level between rapidly growing hepatoma, and regenerating, embryonic and differentiating liver.

The results lead to the conclusion that in the tumors there is an ordered and specific pattern of metabolic and enzymatic imbalance which is also manifested in the cyclic AMP system, carbohydrate, pyrimidine and nucleic acid metabolism and the imbalance is linked with tumor growth rate.

The neoplastic pattern is both quantitatively and qualitatively different from that of the various normal control tissues. A careful examination of the evidence leads to the conclusion that what is important about cancer is ordered, what is not is the random element and the diversity.

ACKNOWLEDGMENTS

The research work outlined in this paper was supported by grants from the United States Public Health Service, National Cancer Institute, Grant Nos. CA-05034 and CA-13526, the Damon Runyon Memorial Fund for Cancer Research, Inc. and Goldblatt Brothers Employees Nathan Goldblatt Cancer Research Fund.

REFERENCES

1. G. Weber. <u>Advances in Enzyme Regulation</u> 11 (1973)
    in press.

2. G. Weber. <u>Gann Monograph</u> 1 (1966) 151.

3. G. Weber. <u>Naturwissenschaften</u> 55 (1968) 418.

4. G. Weber, in: Twenty-Second Annual Symposium on
    Fundamental Cancer Research, ed. R. B. Hurlbert (Uni-
    versity of Texas Press, Houston, Texas, 1969) p. 527.

5. G. Weber and M. A. Lea. <u>Advances in Enzyme Regulation</u>
    4 (1966) 115.

6. G. Weber and M. A. Lea, in: Methods in Cancer Re-
    search 2, ed. H. Busch (Academic Press, New York,
    1967) p. 523.

7. G. Weber. <u>Gann Monograph on Cancer Res</u>. 13 (1972) 47.

8. G. Klein, U. Bregula, F. Wiener and H. Harris.
    <u>J. Cell Sci</u>. 8 (1971) 659.

9. H. P. Morris. <u>Adv. in Cancer Res</u>. 9 (1965) 227.

10. G. Weber and H. P. Morris. <u>Cancer Res</u>. 23 (1963) 987.

11. M. J. Sweeney, J. Ashmore, H. P. Morris and G. Weber.
    <u>Cancer Res</u>. 23 (1963) 995.

12. S. R. Wagle, H. P. Morris and G. Weber. <u>Cancer Res</u>.
    23 (1963) 1003.

13. M. A. Lea, H. P. Morris and G. Weber. <u>Cancer Res</u>. 26
    (1966) 465.

14. C. B. Taylor, H. P. Morris and G. Weber. <u>Life Sci</u>. 8
    (1969) 635.

15. G. Weber, in: Proc. 10th International Cancer Congress,
    Vol. 1 (Yearbook Medical Publishers, Chicago, 1971)
    p. 837.

16. J. A. Ferdinandus, H. P. Morris and G. Weber. Cancer Res. 31 (1971) 550.

17. S. F. Queener, H. P. Morris and G. Weber. Cancer Res. 31 (1971) 1004.

18. G. Weber, M. Stubbs and H. P. Morris. Cancer Res. 31 (1971) 2177.

19. G. Weber, S. F. Queener and J. A. Ferdinandus. Advances in Enzyme Regulation 9 (1971) 63.

20. G. Weber, J. A. Ferdinandus, S. F. Queener, G. A. Dunaway, Jr. and L. J.-P. Trahan. Advances in Enzyme Regulation 10 (1972) 39.

21. G. A. Dunaway, Jr., H. P. Morris and G. Weber. Life Sci. 11, Part II (1972) 909.

22. G. Weber, in: Advances in Cancer Research 6 (Academic Press, New York, 1961) p. 403.

23. H. L. Elford, M. Freese, E. Passamani and H. P. Morris. J. Biol. Chem. 245 (1970) 5228.

24. H. G. Williams-Ashman, J. Janne, G. L. Coppoc, M. E. Geroch and A. Schenone. Advances in Enzyme Regulation 10 (1972) 225.

25. H. G. Williams-Ashman, G. L. Coppoc and G. Weber. Cancer Res. 32 (1972) 1924.

26. G. Weber, S. F. Queener and H. P. Morris. Cancer Res. 32 (1972) 1933.

27. M. J. Sweeney, D. H. Hoffman and G. A. Poore. Advances in Enzyme Regulation 9 (1971) 51.

28. G. Weber, H. J. Hird Convery, M. A. Lea and N. B. Stamm. Science 154 (1966) 1357.

29. M. A. Lea and G. Weber. J. Biol. Chem. 243 (1968) 1096.

30. J. A. Ferdinandus and J. A. Clark. J. Bacteriol. 98 (1969) 1109.

31. D. O. Allen, J. Munshower, H. P. Morris and G. Weber. Cancer Res. 31 (1971) 557.

32. G. Krishna, B. Weiss and B. B. Brodie. J. Pharmacol. Exptl. Therap. 163 (1968) 379.

33. A. Rethy, L. Vaczi, F. D. Toth and I. Boldogh. In this volume.

34. V. Tomasi, A. Rethy and A. Trevisani. In this volume.

35. J. F. Clark, H. P. Morris and G. Weber. Cancer Res. 33 (1973) 356.

DISCUSSION

J. Schultz, Papanicolaou Cancer Research Institute:
Dr. Weber, this is a question that has come up in private
conversation; I'd like to hear from you what the answer
is. Are these slow, intermediate and rapidly growing hepatomas at each stage equally malignant? Do they, on transplantation, metastasize?

G. Weber, Indiana University: Yes, sir. These are
certainly neoplastic cells. If they are in the rat lung long
enough they will kill the animal. Metastatic lesions arise
primarily in the lung, then subsequently they occur in
other organs including the kidneys. There is no question,
that they are neoplastic cells.

M. Chasin, Squibb Institute: You looked for a change
in the K_m and the proportion of the low K_m and high K_m
enzymes with the cyclic AMP phosphodiesterases. Did
you examine adenylate cyclase for the same parameters?

G. Weber: No sir, we have not done it. This is the
incompleteness of the presentation. We might postulate
that there is also a shift in the isozyme pattern in view
of the decrease in glucagon sensitivity of adenylate cyclase
(D.O. Allen, J. Musnshower, H.P. Morris, and G. Weber,
Cancer Res. 31 (1971) 557). However, the decrease
in glucagon response allows other interpretations. But
an isozyme shift could be present, and this would be in
line with our expectations on the basis of the molecular
correlation concept (G. Weber, Advances in Regulation
11 (1973) in press).

G. Krishna, National Institutes of Health: I want
to ask you if you had studied effect of epinephrine on the
adenyl cylase in hepatomas.

G. Weber: No sir, we have not done this. I would
like to examine this because we assume that the glucagon
response is really a liver specific one and the epinephrine
is a non-specific response in this case. Thus, I would
expect that the epinephrine responsiveness would be retained
to the hepatomas.

J. Miller, Irvine: Have you looked at purine metabolism?

G. Weber: No. This is in the works at the moment.
May I say that alteration reported in the literature, e.g.,
those of Glynn Wheeler and others, are in good correlation
with the growth rate of these liver tumors (G.P. Wheeler,
J.A. Alexander, and H.P. Morris, Advances in Enzyme
Regulation 2 (1964) 347).

H. Sheppard, Nutley: I think you demonstrated,
very definitely and convincingly, that the growth rate
of the tumors you examined is definitely linked with these
metabolic shifts. But, as the slides flashed by, it appeared
to me that with many of the slow growing tumors that either
you were not getting a change or in some cases we may
not be dealing with a change from normal to a tumor situation,
but rather just reflecting a rapid growth rate.

G. Weber: No sir. This is not the case. The point
I made and that I would like reemphasize is that no similar
change in isozyme shift occurs in any rapidly growing
control tissues we examined. Here I refer to the regenerating
liver, the differentiating liver in the embryo, or the newborn
liver. The metabolic changes and the imbalance are characteristic of neoplasia. The same type of changes can be detected
also in the slow growing tumor. This was shown for the
phosphodiesterase in the very slow growing hepatoma
47C. I regret that the slide was not up long enough. However,

you may read this in detail in February issue of Cancer
Research (J.F. Clark, H.P. Morris and G. Weber, Cancer
Res. 33 (1973) 356). The results show that in the slow
growing hepatoma the change is already present, indicating
the decrease in the soluble phosphodiesterase activity
and the shift in the isozyme pattern. But these shifts as
well as the imbalance of the opposing enzymes are minor
in the slow growing tumor and the imbalance becomes more
emphasized as you go from the less malignant to the more
rapidly growing tumor. The advantage of examining first
the very rapidly growing tumor is that you know your end-
point and then you can back track from there. In this fraction,
we can diagnose so to speak, the subclinical and very
mild alterations in gene expression. We know which
way we are going and we are in a better position to detect
the minor imbalance of opposing key enzyme metabolic
pathways and shifts in isozyme pattern.

K.S. McCarty, Duke: I wonder if you would care
to speculate on the effect of the increase in the ornithine
decarboxylase activity which might then result in an
increase in the levels of putrescine, spermidine and spermine.

G. Weber: Well, the facts are that on the basis of
the report of H.G. Williams-Ashman, G.L. Coopoc and
G.Weber (Cancer Res. 32 (1972) 1924) there is an increase
in the amount of putrescine which roughly correlates
with the growth rate of these tumors. I suppose you would
expect from the increase in ornithine decarboxylase activity
that the product of the reaction is increased , especially
in the rapidly growing tumors. Indeed, there is a marked
rise in the concentrations of all three polyamines in the
rapidly growing hepatomas.

K.S. McCarty: I was thinking predominantly that
these very basic compounds could perhaps react with
chromatin and perhaps change the transcription.

G. Weber: Yes, of course the reason Guy Williams-Ashman and I looked into this first of all was to examine possible evidence for such effects. Polyamines have been implicated, and I use the word with caution, implicated in growth, in replication, but rigorous proof for mammalian cells has been missing. We postulated that if we examine the activities of some of the key enzymes and the levels of the polyamines, this would put us on to first base to see whether these parameters move in the right direction, that is to say, increase with the rise in tumor growth rate. If the results had been negative, the approach might have been abandoned. Since the results are encouraging, the program will be continued and we hope to gain a deeper insight.

J. Roth, Yale University: I was wondering if you'd care to comment on the relationship of the molecular correlation concept to the heterogeneity of tumor cells, within a tumor. The fact may be that some tumor cells may be growing at a very fast rate and some may be growing at a much slower rate within a single tumor.

G. Weber: This is correct. I'm glad you brought this up. Apparently, when you deal with solid tumors this is a minor and insignificant matter. In working with some of these tumors over a period of nearly 15 years in my laboratories, and in reports from other laboratories, the repeatability of these results has been absolutely remarkable. Working with rapidly growing tumors at one week or at 2 weeks, or at 3 weeks, taking different parts of the tumor, but always selecting the viable portions, the repeatability is remarkable. Now when we put these tumors in tissue culture, we discovered that we can pull out clones that have different growth rates. As you know, 1 gram of tumor contains 200 million cells. Out of these 200 million, as many cells as there are people in this country, there are some that when we clone them exhibit different growth and other properties. Regarding the solid tumor and for 99% of the metabolic pattern this is not recognizable. However, to get to the bottom of this and to examine this more thoroughly we are doing cell hybridization studies with a very slow growing hepatoma (8999) and a very rapidly growing one (3924A) so that we may be in a better position to understand this, including which genome may be predominant and which enzyme program is being read. In conclusion, for practical purposes, the solid tumor poses no problems.

J. Schultz: I'd like to go back to my question. The first impression one gets in your beautiful demonstration is that these are different stages of neoplasia. In other words, are we to gain the impression from what you said that a slow growing tumor on transplantation can slowly kill the animal, a rapidly growing tumor rapidly kills the animal, or does the slow growing tumor become a fast growing tumor, or is this real characteristic of each tumor line which is always slow growing or always fast growing?

G. Weber: I can share with you my thoughts as to how to look at this. First of all, the tumor lines remain fairly stable. This is one of the great advantages of this spectrum. With some exceptions the tumor lines are stable. I assume that the genome contains the potential for rapid growth, as manifested in the most rapidly growing tumor, but the degrees of expression of this neoplastic potential emerge in different degress in the various hepatoma lines, expressed to a minor degree in the slow hepatomas, and expressed to a gradually fuller extent in the more rapidly growing. Finally, there is full-blown expression of neoplasia in the 3924-A and in the 9618-A2 hepatomas, where in a couple of weeks you can get 20 grams of tissue. The same replicative potential resides apparently in most, perhaps in all of our normal cells, but it is kept under an iron law, just as blood coaggula-tion is kept under an iron law; it must not happen. It is a forbidden transition. The various carcinogens can alter gene expression in various degrees and these

different lines represent different degree in the expression
of malignancy. This is on reason for the usefulness of
the hepatoma spectrum because it provides the possibility
of examining the gene expression in its different degrees
in terms of biochemistry. In turn, the key metabolic
alterations should provide attacking points for chemotherapy.
Does that answer you, sir?

C. Moore, Einstein: l'd just like to ask maybe two
questions. One, in view of the fact that you're looking
at glycolysis, you have shown that the level of enzyme
activity for the high K_m enzyme decreases and the
level of the activity for the low K_m enzyme increases.
Does the summation of the activity of the two enzymes
meaningfully change the glycolytic flux or does it remain
the same?

G. Weber: Yes sir. The shift goes from the regulatory
high K_m enzymes to the low K_m enzymes. The sum of
these enzymes, as l showed in one of the slides, is
increased. All the key glycolytic enzymes are increased
many fold and in parallel with the tumor growth rates.
The flux we also measured and we reported (M.J. Sweeney,
H.P. Morris, J. Ashmore, G. Weber, Cancer Res.
23 (1963) 995) that the glycolysis increased parallel
with the growth rate of these tumors. Thus, with the
increase in the key glycolytic enzymes indeed you have
an increase in glycolysis. This was first demonstrated
in slices. Later on, using the in vivo method of freeze
clamping (G. Weber, M. Stubbs and H.P. Morris, Cancer
Res. 31 (1971) 2177) we showed that this increase in
lactate production was present and that it correlated
with growth rate.

C. Moore: Then that flux does go up.

G. Weber: Yes.

100

C. Moore: Is there any change in the localization of the enzymes? Do you have any change in membrane binding, or in the binding to particular material in the cell of the different enzymes?

G. Weber: For the glycolytic ones, we have.

C. Moore: No, especially for the hexokinase, is what I'm getting at.

G.Weber: We have not gone into this but Dr. Weinhouse and his associates in Philadelphia and others have examined this.

S. Strada, University of Texas: Could you give me the evidence that the high K_m form of the enzyme is a regulatory form of the enzyme?

G. Weber: Well, this is in the literature. The high K_m in the case of the glucokinase was reported first by Weinhouse, then later by Weber, by Niemeyer and by Ilyin that the enzyme activity goes down in diabetes and insulin induces the enzyme; this is the enzyme that responds to nutritional and hormonal stimulation. Pyruvate kinase, as we were the first to report, decreased in the diabetic and it was induced by insulin in a dose dependent fashion (G. Weber, M.A. Lea, E.A. Fisher, and N.B. Stamm, Enzymol. Biol. Clin. 7 (1966) 11). We also proved this with anti-insulin serum (G. Weber, Israel J. Med. Sci. 8 (1972) 325). We isolated some of these enzymes and made antibodies against them. These facts seem to be well established.

S. Strada: This then is your premise on which the isozyme shift was based. I was referring to the evidence for the high K_m form of the phosphodiesterase being the regulatory form of the enzyme.

G. Weber: Oh, this is by no means certain yet.

R.Sharma, VA Hospital, Memphis: Have you made
your assays on the total phosphodiesterase activity
of these hepatomas? And if you have, have they increased
as compared to the livers?

G. Weber: I have shown several slides indicating
that the supernatant phosphodiesterase was decreased
in the slow growing hepatoma, and it was very low in
the rapidly growing tumor. These enzyme assays were
done in the supernatant fluid; in these tumors the activity
in the membranes has not yet been assayed. You will
hear later on in this Symposium two papers that involve
assays also in the membrane by Réthy and by Tomasi.

Regulation of Growth Rate, DNA Synthesis And Specific Protein Synthesis by Derivatives Of Cyclic AMP in Cultured Hepatoma Cells

W.D. Wicks, R. Van Wijk[1], K. Clay and C. Bearg
Department of Pharmacology
University of Colorado Medical Center
Denver, Colorado 80220
and
M.M. Bevers and J. Van Rijn
Van't Hoff Laboratory, State University
Utrecht, The Netherlands

ABSTRACT: Analogs of cyclic AMP which are effective inducers of tyrosine transaminase and PEP carboxykinase produce a reversible, dose-dependent inhibition of the rate of growth of cultured Reuber H35 hepatoma cells. The prolongation of the doubling time produced by $N^6,O^{2'}$-dibutyryl cyclic AMP (DBcAMP) leads to a higher percentage of larger cells with correspondingly greater protein content but with the same content of DNA. Studies of the mitotic index and [^{3}H]-deoxyadenosine incorporation in partially synchronized cells revealed that DBcAMP acts primarily by extending the DNA synthetic phase of the cell cycle. The inhibitory effect of the cyclic nucleotide appears to be exercised throughout this phase of the cell cycle and not just at initiation of replication. The effects of DBcAMP on growth and DNA synthesis can be overcome by addition of deoxyribopyrimidine nucleosides suggesting that the cyclic nucleotide may act by interfering with the synthesis of these precursors. The growth of at least one other cultured hepatoma cell line is inhibited by cyclic AMP analogs but another hepatoma line and a normal rat liver line are not affected. Possible explanations for these differences are discussed.

[1] Present address: Van't Hoff Laboratory, State University, Utrecht, Netherlands

INTRODUCTION

Increasing attention has been focused on the role of cyclic AMP in the regulation of cellular growth in the past few years. As evidenced by this symposium, particular interest has been paid to the inhibition of the growth rates of a wide variety of cultured mammalian tumor cells (1-6). The effects of the cyclic nucleotide and its derivatives appear to be quite specific in most (but not all (5)) cases and agents which perturbate the intracellular concentration of cyclic AMP also influence the rate of cellular growth (7,8). The exact mechanism(s) by which growth is regulated by cyclic AMP, however, is not clear in any of the systems investigated to date. DNA synthesis is obviously inhibited ultimately but it is not known whether cyclic AMP acts directly on replication or influences some component of the cell cycle distant from the DNA synthetic (S) phase.

We have found that the growth of the Reuber H35 hepatoma cells in monolayer culture is markedly inhibited by a variety of derivatives of cyclic AMP (9,10). The effect is highly specific for cyclic AMP derivatives and is observed only with those compounds among a series of 6- and 8- substituted analogs which are also effective inducers of tyrosine transaminase and PEP carboxykinase. As will be shown in this report, the growth of the cells is inhibited by a cyclic AMP-dependent prolongation of the DNA replicative phase(S) of the cell cycle. A variety of experiments are provided which indicate that the cyclic nucleotides inhibit overall DNA synthesis and not just initiation of replication. The addition of deoxycytidine, but not cytidine, overcomes the inhibitory effects of cyclic AMP analogs on growth rate and DNA synthesis suggesting that changes in deoxyribopyrimidine nucleotide metabolism may lie at the heart of the action of cyclic AMP.

EXPERIMENTAL

The methods of culturing and handling of the H35 hepatoma cells have been described previously in detail (9-11). The growth medium consists of Eagle's basal medium enriched 4-fold with vitamins and essential amino acids and buffered with tricine at pH 7.4. Fetal calf serum and calf serum were added to 5% and 10% respectively. Under these conditions the generation time for H35 cells is 25-30 hours during exponential growth. The cells are grown in plastic Falcon flasks with a surface area of 25cm^2 at 37° in a dry incubator. Testing for mycoplasma either using growth in enriched broth or autoradiography with [^{3}H]-thymidine has been negative.

The number of cells has been determined either by counting with a hemocytometer after harvesting with 1mM EDTA (9), or by determination of the DNA content by the method of Burton (12). The content of DNA has been found to be invariably 14µg per 10^6 cells even after treatment with cyclic AMP derivatives (9,10). The protein content was measured, after washing the cells twice with 0.9% NaCl, by the method of Lowry et al (13). Incorporation of labelled precursors was measured by the filter paper disc method (14). In the case of DNA synthesis measurements, the TCA step at 85°C was omitted. The suitability of the various labelled deoxyribonucleosides as precursors of DNA was verified by resistance of the acid-insoluble radioactivity to RNase, pronase and alkaline digestion (after reacidification) and its complete sensitivity to digestion with DNase (9).

Partial synchronization of the cells was achieved by a single thymidine (5mM) blockade of log phase cells (9). DNA synthesis was reinitiated by replacing the culture medium with one devoid of thymidine but, in certain instances, containing N^6,0$^{2'}$-dibutyryl cyclic AMP (DBcAMP). Mitotic index determinations were performed after fixation in situ with 10% formalin in a buffered salt solution and staining with Feulgen's stain after washing (15). A minimum of 2,000 cells was scored for mitotic figures.

The various tissue culture materials used in these studies were purchased from Grand Island Biological Co., except in the early studies, for calf serum which was obtained from Biogen Co. and fetal calf serum from Colorado Serum Co. N^6,0$^{2'}$-dibutyryl cyclic AMP was purchased from Boehringer Mannheim. [^{3}H]-leucine (4,5), [^{3}H]-2'-deoxyadenosine (G), [^{3}H]-2'-deoxyguanosine (G), [^{3}H]-2'-deoxycytidine (G) and [^{3}H]-thymidine (methyl) were obtained from New England Nuclear Corporation. The 6- and 8-substituted analogs of cyclic AMP were generously provided by the ICN Nucleic Acid Research Institute in Irvine, California and we would like to thank Drs. R. K. Robbins, M. Stout and L. N. Simon for their assistance.

RESULTS AND DISCUSSION

Figure 1 illustrates a typical growth curve for H35 cells growing under usual conditions.

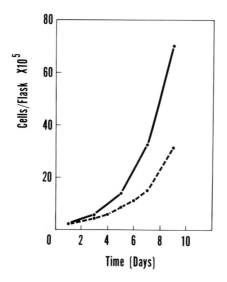

Figure 1. Effects of DBcAMP on the growth of H35 cells. DBcAMP (0.5mM) was first added 24 hours after sub-culturing and the medium was changed every 2 days. Each point represents the average of 3-4 flasks with a standard error of less than 10%. No additions, (——); DBcAMP (---).

Adapted from Van Wijk, et al (10).

Although it does not noticeably influence the attachment of cells to the plastic substrate, DBcAMP was not added routinely until 24 hours after subculture. As can be seen cells exposed to DBcAMP (0.5mM) exhibit a marked lengthening of the generation time. In most cases the cells exposed to DBcAMP continue to grow at a slow rate until other factors restrict their growth and a premature levelling off phenomenon such as seen with transformed 3T3 cells (4) or glioma cells (16) is not observed. Addition of DBcAMP at later intervals also leads to growth inhibition but the effect becomes somewhat less pronounced. Removal of DBcAMP leads to a rapid restoration of the growth rate typical of untreated cells (9). Treated cells can be subcultured after removal of DBcAMP and exhibit normal plating efficiency and growth characteristics. There is no evidence which suggests that exposure to DBcAMP alters H35 cells in other than a transient, phenotypic manner.

Although some toxicity is observed with a wide variety of nucleotides (5'-AMP, cyclic 2',3'-AMP etc.) including DBcAMP in high concentrations in the presence of low levels of calf serum, only DBcAMP and certain other analogs of cyclic AMP (see below) are capable of prolonging the generation time of H35 cells which remain attached to the flask surface in the presence of 10% calf serum (9). For reasons not immediately apparent, under these conditions the non-specific toxic response is not observed (9).

Table I illustrates the specificity of the inhibitory effects of various compounds on the growth of H35 cells. Only analogs of cyclic 3',5'-AMP were capable of reducing the rate of growth of H35 cells and such compounds as buty-rate, 5'-AMP, cyclic 2',3'-AMP, cyclic 3',5'-AMP and prostaglandin E_1 did not significantly affect the growth rate. Among a number of 6- and 8-substituted analogs of cyclic AMP tested, there is a rough correlation between their ability to inhibit growth and to induce the synthesis of tyrosine transmainase and PEP carboxykinase with the exception of the fact that the 6-substituted analogs and 8-NHC_2H_4OH analog lead to rapid cell death (9,11,17). Glial tumor cells are also killed by 8-NHC_2H_4OH cyclic AMP (18), but the basis for this phenomenon is not understood at present.

TABLE I

Effects of Various Compounds on
The Growth Rate of H35 Cells[*]

Compound Added	Concentration	% Untreated Cell Density
DBcAMP	0.5mM	44
3':5'-cAMP	0.5mM	96
	1.0mM	94
2':3'-cAMP	0.5mM	96
	1.0mM	90
5'-AMP	0.5mM	102
	1.0mM	96
Sodium Butyrate	1.0mM	100
Prostaglandin E_1	100µg/ml	100
Prostaglandin E_1 + DBcAMP	100µg/ml 0.5mM	44
8-SH cAMP	0.5mM	64
8-SCH$_3$ cAMP	0.5mM	21

[*]Adapted from Van Wijk, et al (9).

All compounds were first added 24 hours after sub-culturing. Cell densities were determined by counting cells at 6 days. The medium was changed every 2 days and fresh additions were made. Each value represents the average of at least 3 separate flasks and in most cases several more.

The effect of DBcAMP on the growth rate of H35 cells is dose-dependent with a minimum inhibition observed at less than $5 \times 10^{-5}M$ (9) (Fig. 2A). Other analogs of cyclic AMP also exhibit dose-dependent inhibition of cellular growth (17).

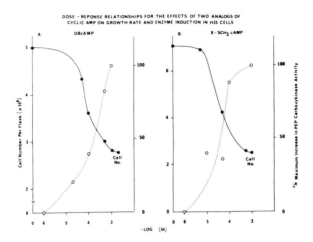

DOSE - REPONSE RELATIONSHIPS FOR THE EFFECTS OF TWO ANALOGS OF CYCLIC AMP ON GROWTH RATE AND ENZYME INDUCTION IN H35 CELLS

Figure 2. In the experiments on growth rate, the analogs were first added 24 hrs after subculture. The medium was changed 48 hrs later and the cells harvested on the day after the medium change. The total DNA content per flask was determined and the number of cells calculated from the known DNA content per cell. Each point represents the average of 3 flasks with a standard error of less than 10%. In the enzyme induction experiments, the analogs were added 7 days after subculture and the cells harvested 5 hrs later. PEP carboxykinase activity was assayed as described previously (11). Each point is the average of 4 flasks with a standard error of 10-15%. $A, N^6, O^{2'}$-dibutyryl cyclic AMP; $B, 8$-SCH$_3$-cyclic AMP.

The relationship between enzyme induction and growth inhibition is further underscored by the correlation between the dose-response characteristics of the two processes with DBcAMP (Fig. 2A) and with 8-SCH$_3$ cyclic AMP (Fig. 2B). The precise basis for the relationship between these processes is unknown at present, but one possible common denominator can be found in the cyclic AMP-dependent protein kinase (19). Indeed, there is a good correlation between the ability of various analogs to induce PEP carboxykinase and tyrosine transaminase (20) and their ability to activate the protein kinases from bovine brain and rat liver (21). At present no evidence is available which demonstrates in a direct manner that protein phosphorylation plays any role in regulating either of these processes. Consequently, the basis for the observed correlation can only be the subject of speculation.

The explanation for the lack of effect of cyclic AMP itself on enzyme induction and growth rate in H35 cells is not clear, but the observed responses are clearly produced only by analogs which mimic the action of the parent compound (9,10,11,17,20,21). The problem may be related to poor transport or rapid metabolism of the free nucleotide. This explanation, of course, could also be invoked to account for the lack of effect of some of the analogs.

There is an effect of cyclic AMP analogs on the morphology of H35 cells, but it appears to be largely indirect (9). Under conditions where the cell density is low, H35 cells tend to be rather large and often exhibit cytoplasmic extensions or processes. As growth progresses and higher densities are achieved, the cells become smaller and more tightly packed and processes cannot be as readily seen (Fig. 3). Treatment with DBcAMP and other active analogs leads to a proponderance of larger cells with prominent nuclei and frequent process formation (Fig. 3). There is, however, no conclusive evidence as yet that this effect is more than an indirect result of the lengthening of the generation time produced by these compounds.

Although the DNA content of H35 cells grown in DBcAMP does not change, the protein content of these cells is considerably increased by such treatment (Table II). In addition, the rate of overall protein synthesis is not reduced by growth in DBcAMP (9). Indeed, it can be calculated from the incorporation data that 30-40% more protein should be synthesized in one generation time with cells grown in DBcAMP if the average rate of protein synthesis does not change and this figure is in excellent agreement with the observed differences in protein content measured chemically (9). Thus, DBcAMP does not inhibit

110

the growth of these cells by way of a major perturbation of protein synthesis.

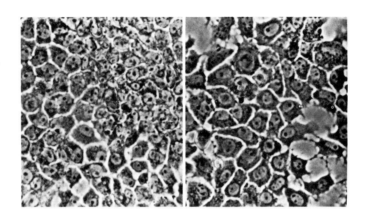

Figure 3. Morphology of H35 cells grown in the absence and presence of DBcAMP. DBcAMP was first added 24 hrs after subculture and the medium with and without DBcAMP was changed 48 hrs later. The cells were photographed 16 hrs later at a magnification of 100x. Left panel, control cells; right panel, cells grown in DBcAMP.

The next experiments were aimed at determining which phase(s) of the cell cycle were lengthened by exposure to DBcAMP. Initially colcemid was employed in an effort to synchronize cells in metaphase, but there was no change in the mitotic index with concentrations of the alkaloid 7 times higher than those which arrest mitosis in HTC cells (17). Consequently, we have made use of the single thymidine blockade technique to partially synchronize cells and then released the block in the presence and absence of DBcAMP (10). The results of such experiments are illustrated in Fig. 4 and they demonstrate that the S phase is rapidly and markedly prolonged by exposure to DBcAMP (10) The main wave of mitoses occurs at 18-20 hours (S+G_2+M interval) after release from a 12, 20 or 36 hour thymidine block with untreated cells. Addition of DBcAMP at the time of release, however, leads to a consistent delay in

TABLE II

Effects of DBcAMP on the Increase in Cell Number, Amount of Protein, DNA and Rate of [3H]-Leucine Incorporation in H35 Cells*

	No. of Cells Per Flask	Doubling Time of Cells (hr)	Protein (μg/10^6 Cells)	DNA (μg/10^6 Cells)	[3H]-Leucine Incorporated (cpm/0.5 hr/cell)
Control Cells	7×10^6	40	300	14	2.7×10^{-3}
DBcAMP-Treated Cells	4×10^6	56	410	14	2.6×10^{-3}

* Taken from Van Wijk, et al. (9).

Cells were grown for 6 days after initial inoculation with 0.6×10^6 cells per flask, and DBcAMP (0.5mM) was first added 24 hours after subculturing. The doubling time of the cells was determined by constructing a growth curve. After 6 days, 6 flasks of each group were used for determination of the initial rate of [3H]-leucine incorporation into protein. For these measurements the medium was changed, and 5ml of growth medium (containing 0.9mM [1H]-leucine), with or without DBcAMP, was added along with 25μCi of [3H]-leucine (36,000 μCi/μmole). The rate of incorporation of [3H]-leucine into protein was linear for at least 90 min. The same flasks were used for determination of the amount of protein per cell. The DNA measurements were performed in several different experiments.

the main mitotic wave until 34-36 hours after release in each case.

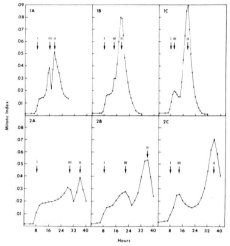

Figure 4. Mitotic index analysis after release of H35 cells from a single thymidine blockade in the presence and absence of DBcAMP. Thymidine (5mM) was added to H35 cells 4 days after subculture for a period of 12 hrs (A), 20 hrs (B), or 36 hrs (C). After removal of thymidine, the cells were placed in medium without (1) or with (2) DBcAMP (0.5mM). At the intervals indicated, the mitotic index was determined. In the figures A, B and C arrows mark the following points: 1) the first increase in mitotic index (used for estimation of the G_2+M interval); 11) the main peak of mitotic figures (used for estimation of the G_2+M+S interval; 111) a small synchronized cell population which appears to represent cells which originated at the G_1/S boundary early after initiation of the thymidine blockade and whose movement through S is also inhibited by DBcAMP (10).

Taken from Van Wijk, et al (10).

Estimates of the length of the other phases of the cell cycle (10) suggested no change in G_2 (the interval between release from thymidine blockade and the first increase in the mitotic index, see Fig. 4), a small increase in M (from the area under the mitotic index vs. time curve for a division wave) and no change in G_1 (obtained by subtraction of G_2, S and M from the generation time) (Table III) (10).

TABLE III

Life Cycle Analysis of H35 Cells Grown in the
Absence and Presence of DBcAMP[*]

Phase of Life Cycle	Duration of Cell Cycle Phases in:	
	Control Cells	DBcAMP-Treated Cells
	Hrs.	
$T^{\dagger}$	30	48
$M + G_2 + S^{\ddagger}$	17.5	36
$M + G_2^{\ddagger}$	7	7
$M^{\S}$	0.6	0.9
$G_2^{\P}$	6.4	6.1
$S^{\P}$	10.5	29.0
$G_1^{\P}$	12.5	12

[*] Taken from Van Wijk, et al (10).
DBcAMP (0.5mM) was added at the time of release of the
thymidine blockade.
[†] Total generation time was obtained from a corresponding
growth curve after release from thymidine blockade.
The number of cells was determined every 6 hrs during
60 hrs. Six flasks were used for each point with a
standard error generally about 5%.
[‡] Measured as time lag after release from the thymidine
block as illustrated in Fig. 4.
[§] Measure from the area under the mitotic index vs. time
curve for a division wave. The figures are the
averages from 3 experiments with a standard error of
approximately 15%.
[¶] Obtained by subtraction of appropriate values.

Thus, it appears that the predominant effect of DBcAMP is exerted on the replication process itself. An estimate of the length of the S phase has also been made from the interval during which [3H]-deoxyadenosine is incorporated after release from thymidine blockade and the values are in good agreement with the mitotic index data (see below and 17). Autoradiographic analysis has confirmed this conclusion by revealing that cells grown in DBcAMP exhibit a much higher percentage of labelled nuclei (60%) than do untreated cells (34%) after pulse-labelling with [3H]-deoxythymidine (17). The observed values are in excellent agreement with those which can be calculated from the respective generation times and the length of S in untreated cells assuming that the increase in generation time is all due to an increase in the length of S. These results provide independent confirmation of the effect of DBcAMP in the overall replication process.

These results are most consistent with an effect of DBcAMP on total DNA synthesis and not just on the initiation of replication. This conclusion is supported by the observation (10) that DNA synthesis is partially inhibited by the addition of DBcAMP to interphase cells within only a fraction (~ 2 hrs) of the total S phase (~ 10-12 hrs) (Fig. 5, curve B).

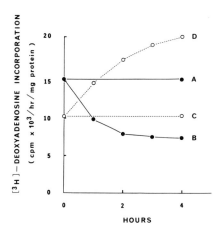

Figure 5. Effect of addition or removal of DBcAMP on [3H]-deoxyadenosine incorporation into DNA in interphase

H35 cells. Cells were grown in the presence (curves C, D) and in the absence (curves A, B) of DBcAMP (0.5mM). The medium with and without DBcAMP was changed on days 2 and 4. Curve A: control cells. Curve B: DBcAMP (0.5mM) was added to control cells 12 hrs after the second change of medium. Curve C: cells grown continuously in DBcAMP (0.5mM). Curve D: cells treated as in curve C were transferred to medium devoid of DBcAMP 12 hrs after the second change of medium (which had contained DBcAMP). DNA synthesis was monitored at the intervals indicated by pulse-labelling for 1 hr with [^{3}H]-deoxyadenosine (1μCi and 0.4μM per flask). Each point represents the average of 3 separate flasks with a standard error of less than 10%. Incorporation of [^{3}H]-deoxyadenosine into DNA is linear under these conditions for at least 120 minutes in untreated and DBcAMP-treated H35 cells.

Taken from Van Wijk, et al (10).

Cells grown in DBcAMP exhibit a reduced rate of [^{3}H]-deoxyadenosine incorporation in spite of the fact that twice as many cells are engaged in replication (curve C). This fact accounts for the lower incorporation in cells exposed to DBcAMP for only 2-4 hours (curve B) in comparison to cells continuously grown in the presence of the cyclic nucleotide analog. Removal of DBcAMP leads to release of the inhibition of DNA synthesis as rapidly as it is instituted (curve D vs. curve B). Once again the higher rate of incorporation 2-4 hours after release is due to the greater percentage of cells in S in the DBcAMP-treated group (curve D) relative to untreated cells (curve A).

These results suggest that DBcAMP rapidly alters the synthesis of DNA such that a new limitation is placed on the process. This limitation appears to be one which is exercised throughout the replication process. Further confirmation of this concept is provided by the fact that the addition of DBcAMP 4 hours after release from a thymidine block exerts a similar rapid inhibitory effect on [^{3}H]-deoxyadenosine incorporation as when the cyclic nucleotide analog is added immediately after release (Fig. 6) (10).

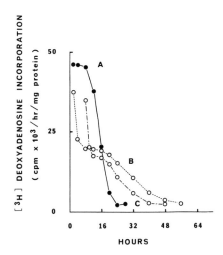

Figure 6. Effect of immediate or delayed addition of DBcAMP on [3H]-deoxyadenosine incorporation into DNA after release of H35 cells from thymidine blockade. Thymidine (5mM) was added 4 days after subculture. After 20 hrs cells were released from thymidine blockade and then incubated without DBcAMP (curve A), or with DBcAMP (0.5mM) added immediately (curve B) or after 4 hrs (curve C). [3H]-deoxyadenosine incorporation was measured as that occurring over a 1 hr interval (1μCi and 0.4μM per flask). The mitotic index curve obtained in this experiment was analogous to that in Figure 4 for cells released without (panel 1B) and with DBcAMP (panel 2B). Each point represents the average of 3 flasks with a standard error of less than 10%.

Taken from Van Wijk, et al (10).

Analysis of the effects of DBcAMP on the incorporation of other [3H]-deoxyribonucleosides (10) has revealed quantitative differences (Table IV). [3H]-Thymidine and [3H]-deoxycytidine incorporation was not as severely inhibited as that of [3H]-deoxyadenosine or [3H]-deoxyguanosine. These results suggested that DBcAMP might be interfering in some way with the formation of deoxyribopyrimidine nucleotide precursors. In fact, it was found that addition of deoxycytidine but not cytidine completely reversed the

117

TABLE IV

Incorporation of [3H]-labelled
Deoxyribonucleosides into DNA in H35 Cells,
Grown in the Absence and Presence of DBcAMP[*]

| [3H]-Precursor | Incorporation in: | | Percent |
	Control Cells	DBcAMP-Treated Cells	Inhibition
	(cpm per 10^4 cells)		
Deoxyadenosine	101	27	73
Deoxyguanosine	61	18	72
Deoxycytidine	61	34	43
Thymidine	1469	634	57

[*] Adapted from Van Wijk, et al (10).

DBcAMP (0.5mM) was first added 24 hours after sub-culturing. The medium with and without DBcAMP was changed on day 2 and day 4. Four hours after the last medium change, the labelled precursors were added. All labelled compounds were added at 1µCi/flask at a concentration of 0.4µM for a 1 hour period. At the time of pulse-labelling, control cultures contained an average of 3×10^6 cells and 360µg protein per 10^6 cells. DBcAMP-treated cultures contained an average of 1.2×10^6 cells and 450µg protein per 10^6 cells. Each value represents the average of 3 separate observations with a standard error of less than 10%.

effects of DBcAMP on growth rate and DNA synthesis (Table V). Deoxyuridine and low concentrations of thymidine also reversed the effects of DBcAMP. These results suggest that formation of deoxyribopyrimidine nucleotides may be inhibited in some way by DBcAMP. Current studies are aimed at analyzing the pool sizes of different precursors of DNA and determination of which of these are subject to regulation.

Deoxycytidine does not owe its ability to reverse the effects of DBcAMP to inhibition of the uptake of the cyclic nucleotide since induction of tyrosine transaminase (in the presence or absence of serum) is not blocked by deoxycytidine (Table VI).

TABLE V

Effects of Deoxyribopyrimidine Nucleosides on the Inhibition Of Growth and DNA Synthesis by DBcAMP in H35 Cells

Compound Added	Concentration mM	Control Cells	DBcAMP-Treated Cells	% Inhibition
1. Growth		(cells x10^6 per flask)		
None		6.5	2.2	66
Cytidine	1	6.2	2.6	58
Deoxycytidine	1	5.8	6.0	0
Deoxyuridine	1	4.9	5.1	0
Thymidine	0.08	4.4	3.4	23
2. DNA Synthesis		(cpm per 10^4 cells)		
None		55	11	80
Deoxycytidine	1	39	40	0
Deoxyuridine	1	32	33	0
Thymidine	0.08	22	17	22

DBcAMP (0.5mM) was first added 24 hours after subculturing and the medium was changed on day 2 and day 4. On day 5 cells were exposed to [^{3}H]-deoxyadenosine (0.6μCi per flask and 0.4μM final concentration) for 1 hour. Each value represents the average of 3 separate observations with a standard error of less than 10%.

TABLE VI

Effects of Deoxycytidine on
The Response of Tyrosine Transaminase
To Dibutyryl Cyclic AMP in H35 Cells

Compound Added	Concentration	Serum	Tyrosine Transaminase Units/mg protein
None		–	53.0 ± 3.6 (4)
Dibutyryl Cyclic AMP	0.5mM	–	125.1 ± 7.1 (4)
None		+	25.7 ± 1.0 (5)
Dibutyryl Cyclic AMP	0.5mM	+	82.7 ± 2.6 (5)
Deoxycytidine	1 mM	+	34.0 ± 1.0 (5)
Dibutyryl Cyclic AMP + Deoxycytidine	0.5mM 1 mM	+	84.5 ± 5.7 (5)

Six day H35 cells were placed in fresh medium with or
without serum or additions. Three hours later the cells
were harvested and assays performed (9,11). The values
are mean ± SE with the number of flasks in parenthesis.

The effects of DBcAMP on the growth of two additional
hepatoma cell lines and one normal rat liver cell line
have also been examined (Table VII). The MH_1C_1 hepatoma
cells (22) also exhibited a prolonged generation time after
exposure to DBcAMP, but neither the HTC hepatoma cells
(23) nor the RLC normal liver cells (24) responded to
DBcAMP. It is of interest in this regard that enzyme
induction by DBcAMP occurs in the MH_1C_1 cells but not in
the HTC or RLC cells (17) (except at massive concentrations
of DBcAMP and then only a small increase in tyrosine transaminase is observed (17,25). These observations provide
added assurance that the inhibition of growth of the H35
and MH_1C_1 cells by DBcAMP is not a non-specific, general
toxic response. The ratio of protein to DNA is also
elevated by DBcAMP, and DNA synthesis is reduced in the
MH_1C_1 cells but not in the HTC or RLC cells.

TABLE VII

Effects of DBcAMP on Growth Rate, Protein Content and DNA
Synthesis in Various Liver and Hepatoma Cell Cultures

	Cell Line	Time of Exposure to DBcAMP	Control Cells	DBcAMP-Treated Cells
1. Doubling Time			(hrs)	
	H35		30	50
	MH_1C_1		50	70
	HTC	5 Days	36	36
	RLC		40	40
2. Protein/DNA			(mg/mg)	
	H35		14.7	19.9
	MH_1C_1		14.1	20.0
	HTC	5 Days	12.5	12.6
	RLC		13.6	14.0
3. DNA Synthesis			(cpm/hr/10^4 cells)	
	H35		15.1	8.9
	MH_1C_1		7.2	4.5
	HTC	4 hours	7.7	7.6
	RLC		7.4	7.2

DBcAMP (0.5 mM) was first added 24 hours after subculture in 1. and 2. and 5 days after subculture in 3.
Three hours later 1.0 µCi of [^{3}H]-deoxyadenosine (1 µM final
concentration) was added to each flask and after one hour
the cells were harvested for assays. Each value is the
average of 5-6 flasks with a standard error of less than
10%.

Although it is tempting to suggest that cyclic nucleotide analogs may act by way of protein kinase-mediated protein phosphorylation, there is no direct support for this
possibility. If a key protein involved in deoxyribopyrimidine nucleotide metabolism was subject either to regulation by phosphorylation (direct inhibition, activation
of an inhibitor or inactivation of an activator) or to
inhibition of its synthesis by cyclic AMP derivatives, then

the inhibition of the growth of H35 and MH_1C_1 cells could be accounted for. The lack of inhibition of the growth rate of HTC or RLC cells could then be ascribed to some defect or alteration in either the protein kinase in these cells or of some component in the system beyond the kinase (the putative key protein?).

Efforts are now under way to identify the precise step(s) regulated by cyclic AMP analogs and to determine directly whether protein phosphorylation plays any role in this process.

REFERENCES

(1)   R. R. Burk, Nature, 219 (1968) 1272.

(2)   M. L. Heidrick and W. L. Ryan, Cancer Res. 30 (1970) 376.

(3)   G. S. Johnson, R. M. Friedman and I. Pastan, Proc. Nat Acad. Sci. (USA) 68 (1971) 425.

(4)   J. R. Sheppard, Proc. Nat. Acad. Sci. (USA) 68 (1971) 1316.

(5)   H. Masui and L. D. Garren, Proc. Nat. Acad. Sci. (USA) 68 (1971) 3206.

(6)   T. J. Yang and S. J. Nas, Experentia 27 (1971) 442.

(7)   J. Otten, G. S. Johnson and I. Pastan, J. Biol. Chem. 247 (1972) 7082.

(8)   J. Sheppard, Nature New Biology, 236 (1972) 14.

(9)   R. Van Wijk, W. D. Wicks and K. Clay, Cancer Res., 32 (1972) 1905.

(10) R. Van Wijk, W. D. Wicks, M. M. Bevers and J. Van Rijn Cancer Res., In press.

(11) C. A. Barnett and W. D. Wicks, J. Biol. Chem., 246 (1971) 7206.

(12) K. Burton, Biochem. J., 62 (1956) 215.

(13) O. H. Lowry, N. J. Rosebrough, A. L. Farr and
      R. J. Randall, J. Biol. Chem., 193 (1951) 265.

(14) R. J. Mans and G. D. Novelli, Arch. Biochem. Biophys.
      94 (1961) 48.

(15) J. Paul, Cell and Tissue Culture (The Williams and
      Wilkins Company, Baltimore, 1970) p. 321.

(16) E. H. MacIntyre, J. P. Perkins, C. J. Wintersgill
      and A. E. Vatter, The responses in culture of human
      astrocytes and neuroblasts to $N^6,O^{2'}$-dibutyryl cyclic
      AMP adenosine monophosphate, J. Cell Sci., In press.

(17) W. D. Wicks and R. Van Wijk unpublished observations.

(18) J. P. Perkins and M. Su, personal communication.

(19) E. G. Krebs in: Current topics in cellular regula-
      tion, Vol. V, eds. B. L. Horecker and E. R. Stadtman.
      (Academic Press, New York, 1972) p. 99.

(20) W. D. Wicks, R. Van Wijk, K. Clay and J. B. McKibbin,
      Advances in Enzyme Regulation, In press.

(21) K. Muneyama, R. J. Bauer, D. A. Shuman, R. K. Robbins
      and L. N. Simon, Biochemistry, 10 (1971) 2390.

(22) A. H. Tashjian, F. C. BAncroft, U. I. Richardson,
      M. B. Goldlust, F. A. Rommel and P. Ofner, In Vitro
      6 (1970) 32.

(23) D. Granner, L. R. Chase, G. D. Auerbach and
      G. M. Tomkins, Science 162 (1968) 1018.

(24) L. E. Gerschenson, M. Anderson, J. Molson and
      T. Okigaki, Science 170 (1970) 859.

(25) R. H. Stellwagen, Biochem. Biophys. Res. Communs.
      47 (1972) 1144.

This work was supported by the Netherlands Organization for the Advancement of Pure Research (Z.W.O.), by Grant AM 16753 from the National Institutes of Health, US Public Health Service, by General Research Support Grant RR 05474 to National Jewish Hospital from the same agency, and by grants from the American Diabetes Association and the General Research Support Program of the University of Colorado Medical Center. We wish to thank Dr. R. Lasher for his assistance with the photographic aspects of this work.

DISCUSSION

J.J. Voorhees, University of Michigan: As I understand
the literature, most individuals have found that cyclic AMP
effects the cell cycle either sometime in G_1 in terms of
the G-S boundary and in G_2. You have pretty clearcut
evidence that you're dealing with the S phase. Would you
want to try to comment on what seems to be a fairly unique
arrangement that you have in your system.

W.D. Wicks, University of Colorado: I know what
you're trying to say. As I tried to indicate in an earlier
slide, we were rather disappointed to find that the effect
appeared to be on the S phase. We would have much pre-
ferred it to be an effect on the commitment of cells to DNA
replication, i.e., G phase, since G_1 is presumably where
most normal cells that are not dividing are located. The
only thing that I can say is that we find that this is the
response to cyclic AMP analogs, and whether it plays any
physiological role or not, I think the phenomenon will allow
us to probe for possible sites by which replication can be
controlled. One suggestion I think comes out of the fact
that some of the hepatoma cells do not respond to cyclic
nucleotide analogs is that there may be multiple sites of
regulation, and maybe the H35 cell line has lost the principal
mechanism which involved the commitment to DNA synthesis
and that perhaps this inhibition of the replication process
is a fail safe mechanism. That's the best I can do.

M. Chasin, Squibb Institute: I was struck by your
slide which has the series of the synthetic cyclic nucleotide analogs. We've studied all those compounds and the
6-thio compound has a unique property that might explain
the zero in your last column. It activites kinase, so you'd

expect it to have some effect on enzyme induction, but it didn't. It's the only one of those compounds that does activate kinase. It doesn't have an effect. It's also the only one of those compounds, and this was found by Dr. Ira Weinryb in our laboratory, that inhibits adenylate cyclase.

E. Smith, Boston University School of Medicine: I wonder if you've looked at the effect of cyclic AMP on the transport of nucleosides.

W.D. Wicks: No, we haven't done this extensively. As I said, (Dr. Van Wijk has done most of these experiments), it appears that there's no effect of dibutryl cylic AMP beyond the uptake or conversion of ^{3}H-Thymidine to ^{3}H-Thymidylate. That's the only one that he has looked at in any great detail.

C. Abell, University of Texas, Medical Branch: Is the tyrosine transaminase specific for tyrosine, or will phenylalanine serve as substrate?

W.D. Wicks: That's a good question. It was shown a number of years ago that phenylalanine would act as a substrate with the liver enzyme, and is a much more specific substrate for tyrosine transaminases. We find that the ratio of activity with the H35 enzyme is identical to that in rat liver.

W. Seifert, Salk Institute, San Diego: Is it known in which phase of the cell cycle that the two enzymes are induced by dibutyryl cyclic AMP?

W.D. Wicks: That's another good question. Unfortunately, we haven't been able to do all the experiments. We have done some preliminary experiments by using a thymidine blockade technique and we've found, and this is extremely preliminary, that the basal activity of tyrosine transaminase markedly rises during the S phase and there's apparently relatively little effect of dibutyryl cyclic AMP.

SOLUBLE AND MEMBRANE—BOUND ADENYLATE CYCLASE OF YOSHIDA
HEPATOMA

Vittorio TOMASI, Antal RETHY[*] and Agostino TREVISANI
Institute of General Physiology
University of Ferrara, Italy.

Abstract: In Yoshida hepatoma cells, adenylate cyclase was
found to be present in the plasma membrane as well as
in the cytosol. The membrane enzyme was sensitive to
epinephrine and fluoride and was very slightly influenced by glucagon, on the other hand the "soluble" enzyme
responded to glucagon better than to epinephrine and
fluoride. The hormone concentrations required for
maximal effect were higher for the tumor than for the
liver enzyme. During tumor growth adenylate cyclase
activity decreased in the membrane and rose in the
cytosol. On the basis of our findings, we propose that
hepatoma cells tend to escape the physiological regulation due either to hormones or to cell to cell interaction.

INTRODUCTION

The external milieu of a tissue cell consists of intracellular spaces and lumens used for supply and excretion,
and of other cells. Therefore two main functions can be
attributed to the plasma membrane: one concerned with
transport and the other with cell contact. Modifications of
composition and structure of cell membrane have been recognized as typical characteristic of cancer cells (1,2).

The study of adenylate cyclase of plasma membrane and
of its hormonal control affords an unique situation in that

---

* Present address: Microbiological Institute of the University of Debrecen, Medical School, Debrecen (Hungary).

an extracellular signal by interacting with the cell surface
transmits its message via production of cyclic AMP to the
cell interior (3).

Moreover the study of adenylate cyclase system may allow
to define, at a molecular level, how the cell membrane is
involved in the control of cell growth. This involvement
has been stressed by the observation that cyclic AMP level
modulates contact inhibition of growth and that a decreased
level of cyclic AMP may be associated with transformation
and increased cell division (4-6).

EXPERIMENTAL

Yoshida ascites hepatoma AH 130, about $20x10^6$ cells in
0.5 ml of ascites fluid at the 7th day of growth, was
injected intraperitoneally in to male Wistar rats weighing
about 200 g. Plasma membranes were isolated by a modification of the method of Ray (7),which has been briefly descri
bed (8) and will be reported in more details elsewhere.
Adenylate cyclase, ATPases and 5'- nucleotidase were assayed
as described previously(8,9).Cyclic AMP-phosphodiesterase
was assayed according to Murray et al. (10).

RESULTS

Hepatoma and liver plasma membranes. Fig.1 illustrates
the distribution of subfractions from hepatoma and liver
plasma membrane along a discontinuous gradient. Three subfractions were separated from hepatoma,having sucrose-
buoyant densities of 1.12, 1.14 and 1.16 g/ml. On the other
hand, from rat liver only two subfractions were separated
having buoyant densities of 1.14 and 1.16 g/ml. It may be
recalled that two subfractions have been isolated from liver
plasma (11) and nuclear membranes (12), from the plasma
membrane of chick fibroblasts (13) and from the plasma
membrane of human blood platelets (14). Three subfractions
have been obtained from plasma membrane of SV 40 virus
transformed fibroblasts and of in vivo growing hamster
tumor cells. From membranes of untransformed cells only two
subfractions were separated (Réthy et al., in preparation).

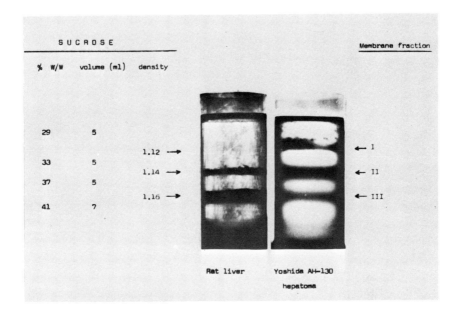

Fig. 1. Distribution of plasma membrane subfractions from rat liver and Yoshida hepatoma in a sucrose density-gradient.

Typical electron micrographs of the plasma membrane subfractions of Yoshida hepatoma are presented in Fig. 2. They appeared to be essentially free from whole mitochondria lysosomes and nuclei. At higher magnification (panels A_1, B_1 and C_1) membrane fractions clearly reveal the trilaminar appearance. Fraction B is probably contaminated by microsomes. Adenylate cyclase had the highest activity in subfraction B and C, while phosphodiesterase activity was distributed in all fractions. A comparison of the heavy subfractions of hepatoma and liver membrane is shown in Table 1. The yield of this fraction was about twice higher from liver than from hepatoma. The gross chemical composition showed minor differences while marked ones could be observed as far as the activity of several enzymes is concerned. In fact 5'-nucleotidase activity was 6 fold, Mg^{2+}- ATPase was about 4 fold and adenylate cyclase was 10 fold lower in

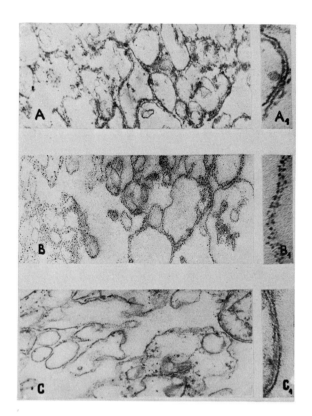

Fig. 2. Electron micrographs of plasma membrane subfractions of Yoshida hepatoma. A, B and C are low magnification micrographs (35,000 x). A_1, B_1 and C_1 are high resolution pictures (220,000 x). A and A_1: subfraction I,
density 1.12; B and B_1: subfraction II, density 1.14; C and
C_1: subfraction III, density 1.16.

hepatoma than in rat liver membrane subfraction. As shown
in Table 2, hepatoma membrane was richer in lipids than
liver membrane, owing to an higher content of glycolipids.

The phospholipid composition is given in Fig. 3. Hepatoma membrane contained several phospholipids (Sp, PS, PI,
PG and PA) in higher amount than liver membrane, in addition
hepatoma membrane included detectable amount of plasmalogens

TABLE I

Comparison of Yoshida hepatoma and rat liver plasma
membranes

	Hepatoma		Liver	
Membrane yield[a]	3.0	(4)	6.5	(30)
mg lipid/mg protein	0.465	(3)	0.411	(6)
μg total Pi/mg protein	12.5	(6)	10.5	(6)
μg lipid Pi/mg protein	10.4	(4)	8.9	(6)
5'-nucleotidase[b]	4.0	(5)	24.1	(7)
Mg^{2+} - ATPase[b]	5.6	(5)	24.1	(7)
Glucose-6-phosphatase[b]	not detected		1.25[e]	
Adenylate cyclase[c]	0.60	(3)	6.49	(4)
c AMP-phosphodiesterase[d]	13.7	(3)	8.5	(5)

a: μg membrane/mg homogenate protein; b: μmoles Pi/ mg
protein/h; c: nmoles c AMP/mg protein/h; d: nmoles adenosine
/mg protein/15 min (substrate was 8×10^{-6} M); e: taken from
Ray (7). Number of experiments are in parentheses.

which according to some workers are typical constituents of
neoplastic cell membranes (15). Rat liver and ascites hepatoma plasma membranes were found to have a different lipid
composition also by Seki et al. (16).

Adenylate cyclase of Yoshida hepatoma and its hormonal
control. The results reported in Table 1 indicate that adenylate cyclase activity of tumor plasma membrane is about
10 fold lower than that of liver plasma membrane. Moreover,
while in liver the ratio between the membrane enzyme and the
homogenate enzyme is about 50, in the hepatoma this ratio
was found to be about 3 (not shown). This was interpreted to
mean that adenylate cyclase might be present in other sub-

TABLE II

Lipid composition of Yoshida hepatoma and rat liver plasma membrane

	mg lipid/100 mg membrane protein[‡]	
	Yoshida hepatoma	Rat liver [*]
Total lipids	46.5 ± 2.4	41.5 ± 1.5
Distribution of lipids:		
Phospholipids	25.5 ± 1.0	22.3 ± 0.4
Neutral lipids	13.1 ± 0.3	16.2 ± 0.6
Glycolipids	7.8 ± 0.3	3.0 ± 0.2

*Data represent the composition of total plasma membranes; for experimental details see ref. (17). [‡]Means of three experiments ± S.E.

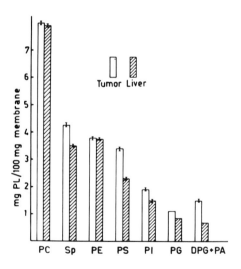

Fig. 3. Phospholipid composition of hepatoma and of liver plasma membranes. For details see Table 2.

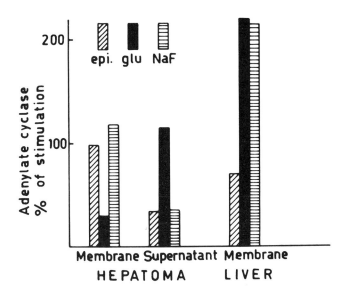

Fig. 4. Hormone and fluoride stimulated adenylate cyclase of hepatoma and of liver. For experimental details see Ref. 8 and 9.

cellular fractions. An examination of the distribution of the enzyme in subcellular fractions of the hepatoma revealed its presence in the cytosol. As shown in Fig. 4, glucagon and fluoride stimulated the enzyme of hepatoma fractions much less than that of liver membrane. When adenylate cyclase activity of other membrane subfractions was studied, it was found that fraction I (see Fig. 1), although having a rather low activity, had an enzyme sensitive to hormones and fluoride. However, since its chemical composition was different from that of liver plasma membrane, and the activity of marker enzymes was low, we did not studied it further. Fraction II, which was found to be contaminated by microsomes, contained an adenylate cyclase activity which was insensitive to hormones and fluoride. As far as soluble enzyme is concerned, as shown in Table 3, we have found an acti̲

TABLE III

Hormone sensitive adenylate cyclase of plasma membrane and
cytosol of ascites hepatoma and rat liver

	HEPATOMA		LIVER	
	membrane	cytosol	membrane	cytosol
Control	0.6 (4)	1.5 (6)	6.5 (4)	0.01 (2)
Epinephrine	1.2* (3)	2.0* (4)	11.0[+] (3)	−
Glucagon	0.8[*] (3)	3.2* (4)	20.8* (3)	−
Fluoride	1.3* (3)	2.0* (4)	20.0* (3)	0.015 (2)

* $p < 0.001$; [*] $p < 0.05$; [+] $p < 0.01$. Activity is expressed
as nmoles/mg protein/h.

vity even higher than that of plasma membrane in the cytosol (Table 3). In contrast to the particulate enzyme, the
soluble one was found to be more sensitive to glucagon than
to epinephrine. The pH optimum (Fig. 5) and the optimal Mg
ions concentration (Fig. 6) are very similar to those repor-

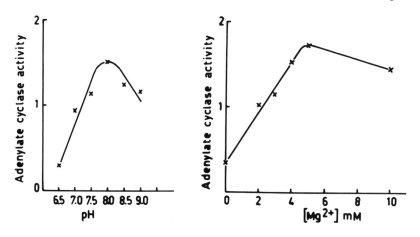

Fig. 5 (left) and 6 (right). The effect of pH (left)
and of Mg ions concentration (right) on soluble adenylate
cyclase activity.

ted for the particulate enzymes of hepatoma and of liver. Fig. 7 shows the hormone concentrations required to obtain

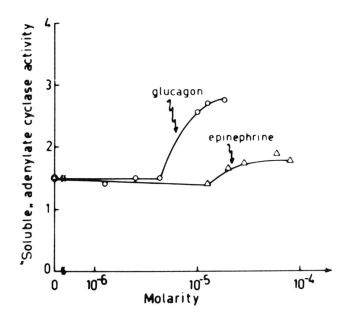

Fig. 7. The effect of epinephrine and glucagon on soluble adenylate cyclase activity.

a maximal stimulation of the enzyme. These amounts appear to be about 5 fold higher than those required for the liver enzyme (18).

To gain more informations about soluble adenylate cycla se, we assayed the enzyme in the membrane and in the cyto-sol of cells grown for different days. The results reported in Fig. 8, indicate that, during the growth, enzyme activi-ty decreases in the membrane and increases in the cytosol, although a quantitative correlation is lacking. The beha-viour of epinephrine-sensitive adenylate cyclase is diffe-rent from that of the glucagon-sensitive enzyme (Fig. 9). This probably means that they are different molecules having a different location in the cell membrane. This view is in accordance with the experiments reported in Fig. 10.

135

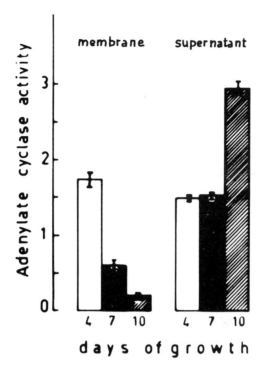

Fig. 8. Adenylate cyclase activity of plasma membranes and supernatant fraction of tumors at different times of growth. Verticals on top of the bars represent S.E. of duplicate experiments on 3 different preparations.

Sephadex G 100 chromatography separated 3 peaks of activity. In the first, adenylate cyclase was insensitive to hormones and fluoride; in the second only fluoride stimulated the enzyme and in the third only glucagon was effective (Table 4). In fraction III glucagon stimulated the enzyme about 10 fold, while it activated the cytosol enzyme about 2 fold. This can be explained by assuming the presence of a soluble inhibitor of the glucagon responsive adenylate cyclase, similar to the macromolecular inhibitor described by Bitensky et al. (19) in the liver.

One important point was to check whether other membrane bound enzymes could be recovered in the supernatant of the

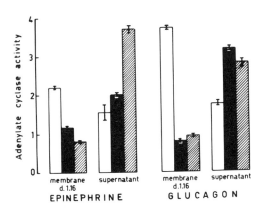

Fig. 9. Epinephrine and glucagon sensitive adenylate cyclase activity of plasma membranes and supernatant fractions of the tumor at different times of growth (4, 7 and 10 days). Verticals on top of the bars represent S.E. of duplicate experiments on 3 different preparations.

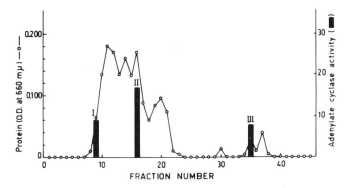

Fig. 10. Sephadex G 100 chromatography of the tumor cytosol. 25 ml of supernatant were placed on a column 3.5x40 cm equilibrated with 0.05 M TRIS–HCl buffer, pH 8.0 containing 0.3 M NaCl. Elution was carried out at 4° with the same buffer. The void volume determined by Blue Dextran corresponded to fraction 12. The bars represent the highest activities.

TABLE IV
The effect of hormones and fluoride on adenylate cyclase
activity of chromatographic fractions

	Sephadex G 100 fractions		
	I	II	III
Control	9.1±0.4	16.8±0.8	6.9±0.3
Epinephrine	11.2±0.5	16.0±0.7	7.0±0.3
Glucagon	9.0±0.5	15.1±0.8	50.9±2.9
Fluoride	10.2±0.6	50.4±2.1	6.5±0.2

Data are means±S.E. of 5 experiments. Epinephrine was 5x
10^{-5} M, glucagon was $1x10^{-5}$ M and fluoride 10 mM. The position of fractions is indicated in Fig. 10.

tumor. We found that the activity of typical membrane—bound
enzymes such as Mg^{2+}— ATPase and 5'— nucleotidase was less
than 10% in the cytosol with respect to the membrane (not
shown).

Cyclic AMP—phosphodiesterase. As shown in Table 5,
phosphodiesterase activity of both supernatant and membrane
of the hepatoma was found to be rather similar to that of
analogous liver fractions. This is in accordance with the
findings of Weiss et al. (20), showing that adenylate cyclase activity of SV 40 virus—transformed hamster astrocytes
was lower than that of normal cells, while no significant
differences in the activity of phosphodiesterase were found
between the two groups of cells. However a phosphodiesterase activity lowered with respect to control, was reported
for an adrenocortical carcinoma of the rat (21).

DISCUSSION

Our observations about a decreased adenylate cyclase
activity and reduced effect of hormones, are in accordance
with recent studies on malignant tissues (4,5,20,22,23).
Makman (23) postulates that an hormone sensitive adenylate

TABLE V

Cyclic AMP—phosphodiesterase activity of hepatoma and liver

	HEPATOMA		LIVER	
	membrane	cytosol	membrane	cytosol
cAMP—phospho-diesterase* A	53	234	33	260
Adenylate cyclase B	0.6	1.5	6.5	0.01
Ratio A/B	88	156	5.1	26,000

*cyclic AMP was 8×10^{-6} M. Activity is expressed as nmoles/mg protein/h.

cyclase is present in malignant cells although its activity is lower than that of cells of nonmalignant origin. According to Makman, adenylate cyclase activity may be enhanced by cell to surface contact or by cell to cell interaction, and this phenomenon may represent a form of self regulation or modulation of the hormonal response by a tissue.

According to Wallach (24) disruption of Ehrlich ascites carcinoma cells leads to the fragmentation of the plasma membrane into diverse vesicle types, each bearing a different complement of the functions of the intact cell surface. If we accept this view, our data showing the presence of adenylate cyclase in the three subfractions of plasma membrane, could indicate that the enzyme is distributed over the entire cell surface. At present it is difficult to evaluate the meaning of this observation. However it may be recalled that differences in the distribution of surface Mg^{2+}— ATPase between normal and neoplastic liver cells have been described (25—27). The enzyme,which in rat hepatocytes is specifically localized at the bile canalicular membrane (2), was found to be present on the entire cell surface of a chemically induced hepatoma (25—27). However this surface alteration does not seem to be specific for all hepa-

139

tic tumors_ since some well differentiated hepatomas have
been found to retain the original distribution of the
enzyme (28). Membrane preparations from hepatomas seem to be
characterized by the presence of low-density subfractions
(2,29).

Several hypothesis can be put forward to account for
the presence of a soluble adenylate cyclase in Yoshida
cells. Two possible ones are: a) the tumoral cells synthe-
tize two different enzymes, a particulate and a soluble
one; b) the membrane-bound enzyme undergoes a partial solubilization during tumor growth or during the procedure of
isolation of membranes. The first hypothesis would better
fit with the fact that soluble and particulate enzyme have
different hormonal sensitivities,as shown in Table 3. Moreover if a solubilization of membrane-bound enzymes would
occur, one would expect to have a situation similar to that
of adenylate cyclase for at least one of the marker enzymes
assayed, namely Mg^{2+}- ATPase and 5'- nucleotidase. In contra
st these enzymes had a very low activity in the tumor cytosol. For what the possible solubilization of the membrane-
bound enzyme is concerned, our data do not permit to exclude
that such a process may play a role in increasing the activity of the cytosol enzyme between the 7th and 10th day of
growth, a period in which the number of cells does not vary
significantly. On the other hand it seems unlikely that
cellular disruption may contribute to the process of solubilization during the exponential phase of growth . Finally
the possibility that our method of membrane preparation
solubilizes particulate adenylate cyclase, may probably be
excluded also in view of the fact that the enzyme is barely
detectable in the cytosol of livers homogenized in the
same conditions used for Yoshida cells (see Table 3).

Pastan et al. (30) have used rather drastic procedures
to obtain a preparation of soluble adenylate cyclase from
an adrenal tumor. Their preparation appears to be different
in several respects from ours. For example it emerged in the
void volume of a Sephadex G 100 column, while our glucagon
and fluoride sensitive enzyme was not excluded by the same

column.

On the basis of the findings of Ganschow and Paigen (31), one could tentatively explain the abnormal distribution of the cyclase by a third hypothesis. These authors found that liver cells of YBR mice lack ergastoplasmic reticulum glucuronidase, but retain the enzyme in lysosomes. This seems to be due to a mutation of a Mendelian gene distinct from the glucuronidase structural gene. The implication of these findings is that the presence of an enzyme in a membrane, is determined by factors other than its primary structure and that separate genes determine these factors (localizing factors). Therefore one could account for the presence of a soluble adenylate cyclase in Yoshida cells, by postulating an alteration of the gene which codify for the synthesis of the localizing factor for adenylate cyclase.

In conclusion, although there are indications that the more anaplastic the cancer is, the lower is the activity of its adenylate cyclase and/or the less it responds to hormones (22,23,32), not all observation fit into this scheme (33-36). This could be due, at least in some cases, to the introduction of artifacts during the procedures of cellular fractionation. Therefore, although our data need to be interpreted with care until they will be integrated with studies regarding modifications of cyclic AMP levels in Yoshida cells incubated in the presence of hormones, we think that they fit into the following scheme. A possible causal relationship between the onset of tumoral growth and cyclic AMP may not necessarily consist in an alteration of the metabolism of the cyclic nucleotide under basal conditions, but mainly in a reduction or in a loss of the physiological regulation of its level. In fact a shift of adenylate cyclase system toward unphysiological or unfavourable positions such as the cell interior, would eliminate or at least strongly reduce, any possibility of regulation either by hormones or by cell to cell interaction.

Abbreviations used: cyclic AMP, cyclic adenosine 3', 5'-monophosphate; PE, phosphatidylethanolamine; PS, phospha

tidylserine; PI, phosphatidylinositol; PC, phosphatidylcho-
line; Sp, sphyngomyelin; PA, phosphatidic acid; PG, phospha
tidylglycerol; DPG, diphosphatidylglycerol.

REFERENCES

(1) D.F.H. Wallach, Proc. Nat. Acad. Sci. U.S.A., 61
(1968) 868.

(2) E.L. Benedetti and P. Emmelot, in: The Membranes, eds.
A.J. Dalton and F. Haguenau (Academic Press, New York,
1968) p. 33.

(3) G.A. Robison, R.W. Butcher and E.W. Sutherland, Cyclic
AMP (Academic Press, New York, 1971).

(4) R.R. Burk, Nature, 219 (1968) 1272.

(5) G.S. Johnson, R.M. Friedman and I. Pastan, Proc. Nat.
Acad. Sci. U.S.A., 68 (1971) 425.

(6) M.L. Heidrick and W.L. Ryan, Cancer Res., 31 (1971)
1313.

(7) T.K. Ray, Biochim. Biophys. Acta,196 (1970) 1.

(8) V. Tomasi, A. Réthy and A. Trevisani, Life Sci., in
press.

(9) A. Réthy, V. Tomasi, A. Trevisani and O. Barnabei,
Biochim. Biophys. Acta, 290(1972) 58.

(10) A.W. Murray, M. Spiszmann and D.E. Atkinson, Science,
171 (1971) 496.

(11) W.H. Evans, Biochem. J., 116 (1970) 833.

(12) D.M. Kashing and C.B. Kasper, J. Biol. Chem., 244
(1969) 3786.

(13) J.F. Perdue and Y.J. Sneider, Biochim. Biophys. Acta,
196 (1970) 125.

(14) A. J. Barber and G.A. Jamieson, J. Biol. Chem., 245
(1970) 6357.

(15) J.K. Selkirk, J.C. Elwood and H.P. Morris, Cancer Res. 31 (1971) 27.

(16) S. Seki, S. Omura and T.Oda, Gann,62 (1971) 89.

(17) A. Réthy, V. Tomasi and A. Trevisani, Arch. Biochem. Biophys., 147 (1971) 36.

(18) G.V. Marinetti, T.K. Ray and V. Tomasi, Biochem. Biophys. Res. Commun., 36 (1969) 185.

(19) M.W. Bitensky, R.E. Gorman, A.H. Neufeld and R. King, Endocrinol., 89 (1971) 1242.

(20) B. Weiss, H.M. Shein and R. Snyder, Life Sci., 10 (1971) 1253.

(21) R.K. Sharma, Cancer Res., 32 (1972) 1734.

(22) P. Emmelot and C.J. Bos, Biochim. Biophys. Acta, 249 (1971) 285.

(23) M.H. Makman, Proc. Nat. Acad. Sci. U.S.A., 68 (1971) 2127.

(24) D.F.H. Wallach, in: The Specificity of Cell Surfaces, eds. B.D. Davis and L. Warren (Prentice—Hall,Inc., New Jersey, 1967) p. 129.

(25) A.B. Novikoff and L.Biempica, Gann Monograph, 1 (1966) 65.

(26) S. Karasaki, Cancer Res., 32 (1972) 1703.

(27) S. Seno, Symp. Cell Chem. Tokyo, 10 (1960) 121.

(28) E. Essner and M.D. Reuber, J. Nat. Cancer Inst., 47 (1971) 25.

(29) N. Chandrasekhara and K.A. Narayan, Cancer Res, 30 (1970) 2876.

(30) I. Pastan, W. Pricer and J. Blanchette—Mackie, Metabol. 19 (1970) 809.

(31) R. Ganschow and K. Paigen, Proc. Nat. Acad. Sci. U.S.A. 58 (1967) 938.

(32) D.O. Allen, J. Munshower, H.P. Morris and G. Weber, Cancer Res., 31 (1971) 557.

(33) H.D. Brown, S.K. Chattopadhyay, H.P. Morris and S.N. Pennington, Cancer Res., 30 (1970) 123.

(34) I. Schorr and R.L. Ney, J. Clin. Invest., 50 (1971) 1295.

(35) C.V. Peery, G.F.Johnson and I. Pastan, J.Biol. Chem., 246 (1971) 5785.

(36) T. Christoffersen, J. Morland, J.— B. Osnes and K. Elgjo, Biochim. Biophys. Acta, 279 (1972) 363.

Acknowledgements: The present work was aided by a grant from the Consiglio Nazionale delle Ricerche to Professor O. Barnabei (Contract 70.0091904). The authors wish to thank Prof. Dr. P. Endes (Institute of Pathology, Medical University of Debrecen, Hungary) for electron microscopical examinations.

DISCUSSION

J. Schultz, Papanicoloau Cancer Research Institute:
Before we start this discussion, I would like to ask a
ground rule question. Now, in this paper we heard the
word stimulation of enzyme activity. In the other paper,
we heard induction of tyrosine transaminases. Now,
we expect that by *induction* is meant a stimulation of
the operon or activation at the level of the DNA in transcription, or translation, on the ribosome. In this paper the
word used is *stimulation*. Now by stimulation, we
usually mean that, in the presence of the enzyme and
substrate in a test tube, that if hormones are added
free of biological material, that you're going to get more
activity per unit of enzyme.

V. Tomasi, University of Ferrara: The concept
of cyclate activation is, if I understood the question,
completely different from the activation via induction
of enzymes. Here we are talking about a modification
of the configuration of an enzyme when the hormone interacts
with the receptor subunit. So actually we are not talking
about a modification of the amount of enzyme, but modification
of its activity. Induction, of course, means that the hormone
must act at the genetic level and increase the amount
of enzyme. That is a completely different question.
Then you need an intact cell. Here we are talking about
isolated plasma membranes which are incubated with
hormone and you see the stimulation of the enzyme,
but the number of molecules does not change, whereas when you are talking about induction, then the number
of molecules is changing.

J. Voorhees, University of Michigan: I think that
you really didn't present any evidence about the number
of enzyme molecules in terms of either more enzyme
or more activity.

W.D. Wicks, University of Colorado: I'm sorry about
the imprecise terminology. This has been a continuing
battle between microbiologists and people who work with
eukaryotic systems. We do not mean by induction that
you're necessarily influencing the genetic apparatus.
We in fact believe that cyclic AMP acts at the level
of translation, in the same way that Dr. Gill talked about
the induction of steroidogenesis of the adrenal cortex,
and we don't think that in the case of these two enzymes
that transcription was involved.

V. Tomasi: I agree with Dr. Wicks.

H. Baer, University of Alberta; Canada: Which
method did you use for adenyl cyclase assay? Have you
made any special effort in this particular and unusual
case to verify cylic AMP formation?

V. Tomasi: Yes. We used a modification of the method
of of Martinetti *et al.*, and 2 dimensional paper chromatography
with some modification, for instance, inclusion of an ATP
regenerating system and other small variations.

H. Baer: Thank you. Have you assayed adenylate
cyclase also in the crude homogenate of Yoshida hepatoma,
or only in the purified fractions?

V. Tomasi: I have also assayed adenylate cyclates
in the crude homogenate.

H. Baer: With respect to ATP'ase in soluble cyclases,
have you measured any ATP'ase contamination, particularly
after gel filtration?

V. Tomasi: The adenyl cyclase is little contaminated with ATP'ase. As a rule, for example, tumor membranes have an activity, as showed before, of about 5 micromoles/milligrams/hour. Now this activity in the supernatant is about of the order of one tenth, one hundredth less. These are very low ATP'ase activities in the supernatant.

Klein, New York University: I was wondering whether at the same time you were demonstrating a loss of the membrane activation by hormones, and a decrease in enzyme activity, if you also measured fluoride stimulatable activity with your membrane cyclase at the time that it was losing activity. Was there also a loss of fluoride stimulatable activity?

V. Tomasi: I showed in the table that the membrane bound enzyme was activited by fluoride as it was by epinephrine. The soluble enzyme was much less activited by fluoride, but I'm talking about the total homogenate. But when you measure the fraction by Sephadex G100, then you can get a fraction which is about threefold stimulated by fluoride.

Klein: I think you demonstrated with your growing cells, that there was a loss of membrane responsiveness; the membrane enzyme lost its responsiveness to epinephrine and to glucogon. The enzyme activity was there. What I'm asking is was there still fluoride stimulatable activity in the same preparation?

J. Voorhees: It seems to me that on one of the slides you showed that there was activation by glucogon and not by fluoride.

V. Tomasi: The problem is that when one takes the total supernatant, or cytosol on a Sephadex G-100 column, one gets three fractions, but one is not stimulated at all, either by hormone or by fluoride. Then you get another fraction which is stimulated only by fluoride, and still another one which is stimulated only by glucogon.

J. Voorhees: It's this last thing that I find rather interesting. You have an explanation for the stimulation by glucagon or fluoride?

V. Tomasi: There's a rather lot of trouble explaining why fluoride stimulates adenylate cyclase, and, of course, it does so only with isolated particles, not within that cell. There are a lot of suggestions regarding the fact that fluoride probably acts by removing an inhibitor of adenylate cyclase. At least this is the idea of people working with particulate adenylate cyclase. Now the problem here is more complicated of course, because you still get fluoride stimulation, unless the inhibitor goes into the fraction where you get activation by fluoride, namely in fraction two. And if this inhibitor doesn't go in fraction three, then of course, you don't get any stimulation by fluoride.

Klein: The slide I was referring to was Fig. 9. The slide demonstrated that both with epinephrine and glucagon, the adenylate cyclase activity decreases. What I'm questioning is, at the same time that you see a decrease in this activity, did you look for fluoride stimulated activity in the membrane preparation?

V. Tomasi: Yes, we looked, and fluoride stimulated activity at that time it was very similar to this one. Of course, the number, the maximum activity was changing but the pattern was very similar to this one.

J. Fessenden-Raden, Cornell University, Ithaca: How did you homogenize your cells?

V. Tomasi: I used a Dounce homogenizer and, usually I used about 40 strokes with a tight pestle and about 20 with a loose one, but you have to use a Dounce homogenizer.

J.F-Raden: Secondly, could you give us the lipid content in your soluble adenylate cyclase?

V. Tomasi: We did not look at the lipid content.

J.F-Raden: Have you done a total phosphate determination?

V. Tomasi: No, we did not determine the soluble phosphate.

J.F-Raden: Have you taken any electron microscope pictures of your soluble fraction?

V. Tomasi: No, we didn't; but if you are thinking about the fact that we can have very small particles coming from the membrane like in Pastan's preparation, then I think that this is very unlikely because Pastan's preparation is composed, if I recall, of very small vesicles of very high molecular weight, about 7 million, and is completely excluded by a Sephadex G100 column, while with our cyclase, only one peak goes into the void volume but glucogon sensitivity and fluoride sensitivity are included. So I am thinking really of a free enzyme, not bound to any membrane particles.

J.F-Raden: I don't think this is quite enough and I would suggest perhaps doing the other assays for membranous material.

V. Tomasi: You are correct.

J.F-Raden: Well, having worked in the mitochondrial field for many years now, I've seen soluble oxidative phosphorylation postulated and die many times, and I think that these are very important controls that should be done before you start postulating that it really is a soluble enzyme.

V. Tomasi: That is a first approach.

J. Voorhees: In relationship to that, I think what she means is perhaps if you were to spin your supernatants very, very hard, perhaps 250,000 x g, then concentrate whatever is there, and then imbed that, then look at that in the electron microscope and find out if perhaps there is something floating around that even in a dilute solution that you couldn't see with negative staining. This might not be a bad idea.

V. Tomasi: Maybe, but I think it is unlikely.

J.F-Raden: I might add to this that even that speed centrifugation might not even be enough.

J. Voorhees: Right. Maybe even a half a million x g!

G. Krishna, National Institutes of Health: It looks from your Sephadex elution pattern, that this glucogen sensitive, soluble cyclase has a molecular weight of about 10 to 20 thousand. Have you calculated it?

V. Tomasi: Yes, it should be 30 to 40 thousand, I think. We did not make careful analyses of this. We are now, and we have a lot of experimental progress. Our idea when we did these experiments was just to exclude the possibility that we were dealing with a small fragment of membrane. And since the soluble preparation goes into the column, we thought that we were not dealing with a small fragment of membrane.

G. Krishna: Did you use $ATP^{32}P$ for these assays and check the cyclic AMP by crystallization?

V. Tomasi: Yes, but we used $ATP^{14}C$ not $ATP^{32}P$.

*A. Wollenberger, Academy of Science of the G.D.R.,
Berlin:* Since this meeting is a sequel of the protein phosphorylation symposium, may I just call attention to a subtle
distinction between the terms enzymes "activation" and
"stimulation" that has become customary in designating
increases in enzyme activity, depending on whether the
enzyme protein is being phosphorylated or is not.
By activation, we understand an increase in enzyme activity
due to covalent modifications, for example phosphorylation,
while by enzyme stimulation is meant an increase in
enzyme activity due to increased substrate availability
or other allosteric transitions. So it might be a good
idea if we stuck to this terminology. But I also have
a question, and this concerns your marker enzymes
for the plasma membranes. Wouldn't the magnesium dependent
sodium and potassium stimulated ATP activity be a more
characteristic enzyme for the plasma membrane than just
the magnesium ATP'ase?

V. Tomasi: Well, that has been done and it correlates
very well, that is, we got sodium and potassium ATPase
activity in the same fraction, the highest activity in the
same fraction we are talking about.

A. Wollenberger: Mg ATPase is also present in intracellular structures.

V. Tomasi: Yes, Mg ATPase is not as good as sodium,
potassium ATP'ase.

Z. Brada, Papanicolaou Cancer Research Institute:
I would like to ask about one thing. The problem is that
many ascites tumors have a very high content of dead
cells. Some ascites tumors have only 1 to 2 per cent,
but in some tumors, I'm not sure about Yoshida hepatoma,
the content of dead cells in vivo is very high, about 40
per cent, and the amount increases during the growth
of tumor. What is the situation with your tumor?

V. Tomasi: The Institute of Pathology of Florence told me that the amount of dead cells, until the seventh day, is very low, with respect to the total amount of cells. Then you may be right, from when we are at the tenth day or so of growth, necrosis could be a problem. But you know we just give our data relating to cell grown from 3 to 7 days, thus these are in the early stage of growth.

ABNORMAL DISTRIBUTION OF ADENYLATE CYCLASE IN

NEOPLASTIC CELLS

A. Réthy, L.Váczi, F.D. Tóth   and   I.   Boldogh

Medical University of   Debrecen,   Microbiological
Institute,   DEBRECEN 12. HUNGARY.

SUMMARY

The distribution of enzymes adenylate cyclase
and cyclic AMP phosphodiesterase has been investigated
in plasma membrane subfractions /subunits/ and in supernatants /1o5.ooo g_{av}/ of cells transformed by   simian virus 40 and Rauscher leukemia virus.

All transformed cells have a hormone-and fluori-
de-sensitive adenylate cyclase in their supernatant
fractions, which do not react to prostaglandins; con-
versely only in traces has been found this enzym in supernatant of normal cells.

Three plasma membrane subfractions have been
found in the virus transformed cells, in contrast
from normal cells two subfractions could be prepared.
Properties of these subfractions were demonstrated.

All the three plasma membrane subfractions of
transformed cells ascertained a hormone /epinephrine,
glucagon/ - sensitive adenylate cyclase activity,
whilst the normal cells contained it only in one subfraction / d 1.16/ .

The activities of hormone sensitive adenylate
cyclase were transferred to lighter membrane subfractions after transformation.

Hormonal responsiveness and stimulation by
prostaglandins of adenylate cyclase were dependent on

transforming agents /DNA or RNA virus/ and also on the growing of tumor cells either <u>in vitro</u> or <u>in vivo</u>.

Cyclic AMP phosphodiesterase activity has been found in all subfractions of membranes in normal and also in transformed cells. It changed after transformation depending on transforming agents.

INTRODUCTION

Intracellular level of cyclic $3',5'$,-adenosine monophosphate /cyclic AMP/ is controlled primarily by the activity of adenylate cyclase and cyclic $3',5'$ – adenosine monophosphate phosphodiesterase /cyclic AMP PDE/, the first being membrane – bound and the second partly particulate and partly soluble /1/.

Tumor cells differ from the corresponding normal ones in structural organization and function of their membranes /2.–5./. Thus abnormalities in cyclic AMP metabolism after neoplastic transformation may, in part, be explained as specific characteristics of transformed cells /6.–10./

In the past few years considerable interest has been focused on the study of plasma membranes isolated from transformed cells /11–14/. However, there are very few data referring to the distribution of hormone-sensitive adenylate cyclase system and to the cyclic AMP PDE in tumor cell membranes. Data relating to the distribution of these enzymes in the plasma membrane subfractions are completely lacking. Therefore it seemed of interest to investigate the latter question all the more as the interpretation of lipoprotein subfractions /subunits/ of membranes gives a new approach to the elucidation of the plasma membranes structural organization /15., 16/.

The necessity of dealing with these questions is stressed by the role of cyclic AMP in regulation of morphology and growth of transformed cells / 17., 18./.

In the course of our investigations the method of Ray was used /19/, modified and recently described by us /20/ for the preparation of plasma

membrane subfractions of cells transformed by oncogenic
viruses. Their gross chemistry and the distribution of
hormone-sensitive adenylate cyclase and cyclic AMP
PDE activity were compared to the corresponding data
of normal cells. Following our earlier investigations
concerning Yoshida hepatoma /21/ the characteristics
of soluble adenylate cyclase were studied in virus
transformed cells.

EXPERIMENTAL

Tumor and transplantation :

a/ Simian virus 40   /SV 40/ tumor was induced and
serial transplantation was performed in hamster
as described by Sabin and Koch /22./, by using
SV 40 strain 777 /obtained from Prof.A.B.Sabin/.
The cloned cell line and cultivation was made
by method of Géder et al /23./. In vivo implants were used after 28 days of transplan-
tation.For control the normal hamster embryo
/BH/ fibroblasts were employed.

b/ Rauscher leukemic spleen of BALB/c mice was
produced as described by Tóth et al /24/. The
spleens were used for experiments after 14 days
of infection. The Rauscher leukemia virus /RLV/
was obtained from Prof. V.M. Bergolts /Gertsen
Institute for Oncology, Moscow/.
Normal spleen of BALB/c mice was used as
control.

For the other methods see legends of PLATES, Tables
and Figures.

Express of enzymes activity :

Activity of adenylate cyclase is expressed as picomoles
cyclic AMP /mg protein/15 min ; activity of cyclic AMP
PDE is expressed as nanomoles adenosine/mg protein/ 15
min.

As for to others see the legends.

RESULTS

Characterization of plasma membrane subfractions.

Electron micrographs of thin section of plasma membrane subfraction of normal and Rauscher leukemic spleen of mice are shown in PLATE I, and those of normal and SV 40 transformed hamster cells in PLATE II. The low magnification micrographs show the membrane sheets interconnected by junctional complexes and a large number of vesicles in all subfractions. The subfraction of transformed cells at density /d/ 1.12 hardly ever contains any nexal form, which is primarily characteristic of the heavy subfraction of normal cells at d 1.16.

The high magnification pictures clearly demonstrate the unit membranes in all the three subfractions of transformed cells.

Explanation of PLATE I

Electron micrographs of thin section of plasma membrane subfractions of normal /b= d 1.14; c and c_1 = d 1.16/ and Rauscher leukemic spleens /A and A_1 = d 1.12 ; B and B_1 = d 1.14 ; C and C_1 = d 1.16/ of BALB/c mice. Electronmicroscopy was performed by the method of Pohl et al /25/. Observations were made with a TESLA BS 513 A electronmicroscope. Magnifications : b, c, A, B, C : 35ooo x ; B_1 : 22oooo x ; c_1, A_1, C_1 : 11oooo x.

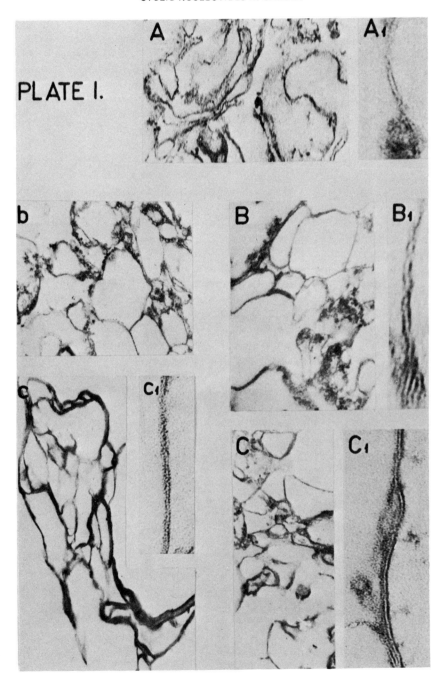

PLATE I.

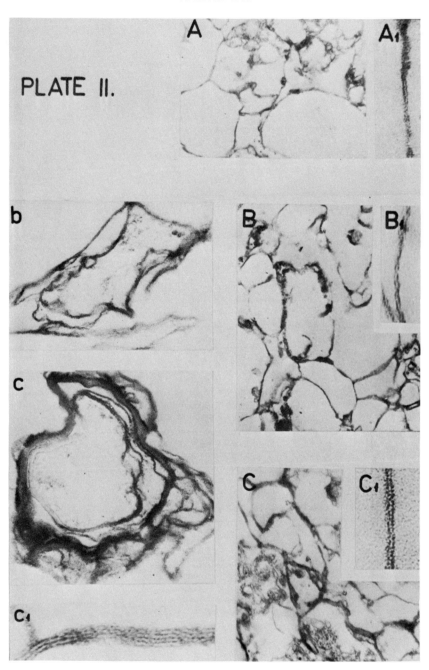

PLATE II.

Explanation of PLATE II

Electronmicrographs of thin section of plasma membrane subfractions of normal /b = d 1.14 ; c and c_1 = d 1.16/ and SV 40 transformed /A and A_1 = d 1.12 ; B and B_1 = d 1.14 ; C and C_1 = d 1.16/ BH fibroblasts.

As for to others see PLATE I.

Magnifications : b, c, A, B, C : 35000 x ; A_1, B_1, C_1 and c_1 : 11oooo x.

Table 1 and Table 2 show the characteristic data of these membrane subfractions.

It should be pointed out that the typical plasma membrane enzym, the 5'-nucleotidase was 11-21 fold higher in membrane subfractions as compared with the homogenate in transformed cells. The activity of the other membrane enzyme i.e. /Mg^{2+}, Na^+, K^+/ - ATPase, was found to be nearly two fold higher in lightest subfractions /d 1.12/ than in subfraction at d 1.16, in both transformed cells. The increased activity of this enzyme was 10.5 - 22.5 fold in SV 40 transformed cells, and 5.5 - 10 fold in Rauscher leukemic spleens as compared with the homogenate. Activity of both marker enzymes showed a decreased value in membranes as opposed to normal cells.

TABLE 1

Properties of membrane subfractions prepared from Rauscher leukemic spleens of BALB/c mice

DATA OF NORMAL SPLEENS ARE GIVEN IN PARENTHESIS

	HOMOGENATE		PLASMA MEMBRANE SUBFRACTIONS					
			d. 1.12		**d. 1.14**		**d. 1.16**	
µg protein/mg total protein	—		6.0	(—)	4.8	(3.1)	3.5	(5.1)
mg lipid/mg protein	—		0.566	(—)	0.525	(0.496)	0.498	(0.435)
5'– NUCLEOTIDASE[a]	0.2	(0.3)	4.3	(—)	2.9	(2.3)	4.1	(9.2)
(Mg^{2+}, Na^+, K^+) ATPase[a]	0.9	(0.8)	9.0	(—)	4.3	(9.1)	4.8	(7.8)
ADPase[a]	0.2	(0.3)	0.0	(—)	0.0	(0.0)	0.0	(0.0)
CYTOCHROM OXIDASE[b]	33.0	(25.0)	0.0	(—)	0.0	(0.0)	0.0	(0.0)
RNA (µg/mg protein)	136.0	(103.0)	15.0	(—)	9.0	(5.0)	8.0	(6.0)

[a] µmoles Pi/mg protein/h
[b] nanomoles cytochrom c/mg protein/min

Preparation of plasma membrane subfractions was performed as previously described /20/. Enzymes activities were assayed according to published procedures : 5'- nucleotidase, Emmelot and Bos /26/ ; ATPase and ADPase, Emmelot et al /27/; cytochrom oxidase, Cooperstein and Lazarow /28/. RNA was assayed with the orcinol reagent /29/. Extraction, purification, and determination of lipids was described by us /30/.

The presented values are an average of 4-6 determinations.

TABLE   2

Properties of membrane subfractions prepared from
SV 40 transformed BH fibroblasts

DATA OF NORMAL BH FIBROBLASTS ARE GIVEN IN PARENTHESIS

| | HOMOGENATE | | PLASMA MEMBRANE SUBFRACTIONS | | | | | |
			d. 1.12		d. 1.14		d. 1.16	
µg protein/mg total protein	—		7.2	(—)	4.3	(3.7)	3.9	(3.3)
mg lipid/mg protein	—		0.528	(—)	0.491	(0.446)	0.427	(0.409)
5'−NUCLEOTIDASE[a]	0.3	(0.6)	4.9	(—)	3.4	(9.3)	5.1	(13.5)
(Mg^{2+}, Na^+, K^+) ATPase[a]	0.5	(0.4)	12.3	(—)	8.7	(12.5)	5.3	(14.1)
ADPase[a]	0.4	(0.4)	0.0	(—)	0.0	(0.0)	0.0	(0.0)
CYTOCHROM OXIDASE[b]	18.0	(15.0)	0.0	(—)	0.0	(0.0)	0.0	(0.0)
RNA (µg/mg protein)	116.0	(125.0)	19.0	(—)	17.0	(9.0)	9.0	(7.0)

[a] µmoles Pi/mg protein/h
[b] nanomoles cytochrom c/mg protein/min

For the methods see Table 1.
The presented values are an average of 4 - 6 determinations.

The lighter subfractions were richer in lipids versus
heavy subfractions /d 1.16/.

The investigated subfractions contained RNA which
was resistent to digestion by RNAse.

Absence of mitochondria was confirmed by a loss of
activity of cytochrom oxidase.

161

Adenylate cyclase and its hormonal control.

Table 3 and Table 4 show the basal adenylate cyclase activity of transformed cells.

TABLE 3

Adenylate cyclase activity in spleens of normal and Rauscher leukemic BALB/c mice

PERCENTAGE OF CONTROL VALUES ARE GIVEN IN PARENTHESIS

CELLS	HOMOGENATE	SUPERNATANT ($105000g_{av}$)	PLASMA MEMBRANE SUBFRACTIONS		
			d 1.12	d 1.14	d 1.16
NORMAL	106 ± 6 (100)	TR	—	142 ± 15 (100)	1161 ± 72 (100)
RAUSCHER VIRUS INFECTED	27 ± 2 (26)	54 ± 4	247 ± 22	358 ± 40 (252)	737 ± 57 (63)

MEANS OF SIX OBSERVATIONS ± S.E.

Adenylate cyclase activity was assayed according to Marinetti **et al** /31/, with some modifications /32/. Incubation medium contained in a final volume of 0.5 ml : 50 mM TRIS - HCl, pH 8.0 ; 0.6 mM ATP-8-C^{14} /o.5 µCi/,RCC Amersham, England /Sp ac 52 mCi /mmole/ ; 4 mM MgCl$_2$; 10 mM aminophylline ; 50 µg bovine serum albumin ; ATP - regenerating system : 15 mM creatinphosphate and 10 IU creatin - phosphokinase ; 80 - 100 µg of proteins. Incubation was carried out for 15 min at 37°. Reaction ran linearly for at least 15 min and was proportional to the amount of fraction used within loo µg protein.

TABLE 4

Adenylate cyclase activity in normal and SV 40 transformed   hamster   embryo   fibroblasts

PERCENTAGE OF CONTROL VALUES ARE GIVEN IN PARENTHESIS

CELLS	HOMOGENATE	SUPERNATANT $(105000g_{av})$	PLASMA MEMBRANE SUBFRACTIONS		
			d 1.12	d 1.14	d 1.16
NORMAL	90±8 (100)	TR	—	TR	462±38 (100)
SV$_{40}$ TRANSFORMED:					
IN VITRO	78±7 (87)	34±4	20±3	44±4	116±18 (25)
IN VIVO IMPLANT	81±8 (90)	42±3	38±4	45±3	307±25 (66)

MEANS OF SIX OBSERVATIONS ± S.E.

For legend see Table 3.

Three important points may be underlined from
these tables:

a/ in supernatant fractions of normal cells adenylate
cyclase activity can be found only in traces, while
the transformed cells contain the enzyme activity
also in soluble   form ;

b/ no significant differences in activity of adenylate
cyclase were observed in homogenate of SV 40 transformed cells as compared with the normal ones,
whereas a significant decreased enzyme activity
appeared in membrane subfractions ad d 1.16, which
was higher in cultured cells than in their in vivo
implants.
On the basis of similar comparisons a decreased activity of the enzyme could be demonstrated in
spleens of mice   infected by RLV.

c/ in all the three membrane subfractions of cells
transformed by oncogenic viruses a hormone-sensitive

163

adenylate cyclase activity was found. In contrast, it was observed only in one subfractions in corresponding control cells / d 1.16/, /see also Fig.1/.

The hormone, fluoride, and prostaglandin sensitivity of adenylate cyclase are shown in Fig. 1 and Fig.2. It should be emphasized :

a/ response to epinephrine decreased and was transferred to lighter subfractions in Rauscher leukemic spleens. The same transferring was observed in hamster cells transformed by SV 40, however response to epinephrine was more enhanced than in the control;

b/ the appearing response to glucagon in leukemic spleens showed an abnormality. It did not decrease in the cells transformed by SV 40, however it was transferred to subfraction of d 1.14 in in vivo implant;

c/ stimulation by fluoride - in general - in lightest subfraction was most expressive;

d/ one of the most striking effects of PGE_1 and $PGF_{2\alpha}$ was that their stimulability in cultured cells transformed by SV 40 could not be observed; in contrast, the in vivo implants definitely reacted to prostaglandins.

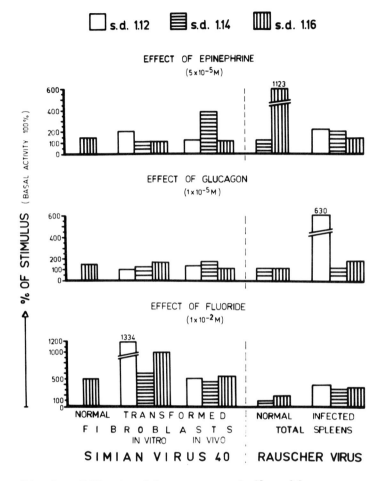

Fig.1. Effect of hormones and fluoride on adenylate cyclase activity in membrane sub-fractions of cells transformed by oncogenic viruses. The bars represent means of four determinations. For others see Table 3.

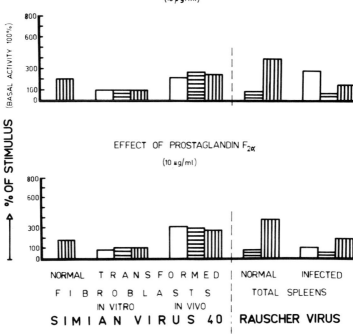

Fig.2. Effect of prostaglandins on adenylate cyclase activity in membrane subfractions
of cells transformed by oncogenic viruses.
The bars represent means of four determi -
nations.

As for to others see Table 3.

Fig 3 indicates the difference between the normal
spleens of mice and those infected by RLV at the concentration to get a maximal stimulation of adenylate
cyclase. In respect of epinephrine and glucagon a similar phenomenon was observed in Yoshida hepatoma as
compared to normal rat liver /21/

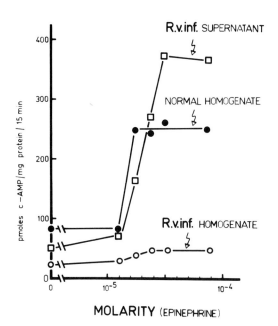

Fig. 3. Effect of epinephrine on adenylate cyclase activity in spleens of normal and Rauscher leukemic BALB/c mice.

Results are means of three observations.

Cyclic AMP phosphodiesterase.

Table 5 and Table 6 show the activity of cyclic AMP PDE of cells transformed by oncogenic viruses. An activity of enzyme was found in all the three membrane subfractions of transformed cells. Its activity was 3.4 fold higher of control values in membrane sub-fraction at d 1.16 of Rauscher leukemic spleens, while a decreased activity was observed in hamster cells transformed by SV 40. The enzyme showed a decreased activity in homogenate and supernatant of both transformed cells, as opposed to normal ones.

TABLE 5

Cyclic AMP phosphodiesterase activity in spleens of
normal and Rauscher leukemic BALB/c mice

CELLS	HOMOGENATE	SUPERNATANT $(105000g_{av})$	PLASMA MEMBRANE SUBFRACTIONS		
			d 1.12	d 1.14	d 1.16
NORMAL	5.6±0.4 (100)	57.1±5.1 (100)	—	TR	3.5±0.2 (100)
RAUSCHER VIRUS INFECTED	3.8±0.3 (68)	20.9±1.2 (37)	8.6±0.4	4.1±0.3	11.8±0.8 (340)

PERCENTAGE OF CONTROL VALUES ARE GIVEN IN PARENTHESIS
MEANS OF SIX OBSERVATIONS ± S.E.

Cyclic AMP PDE activity was assayed as described by Murray et al /33/, with the next modification : incubation medium contained in a final volume of 0.3 ml : 50 mM TRIS-HCl, pH 7.4 ; 10 mM $MgCl_2$; 2 mM cyclic AMP; o.2 µCi H^3-cyclic AMP /sp ac 25 Ci/mmole, RCC, Amersham, England/ and 50-80 µg of protein. The reaction mixtures were incubated at 30⁰ for 15 min, and it was stopped by immersing the tubes in boiling water for 3 min. Then the tubes were cooled and reincubated by adding 25 µg Crotalus adamanteus venom.

TABLE 6

Cyclic AMP phosphodiesterase activity in normal and SV 40 transformed hamster embryo fibroblasts

PERCENTAGE OF CONTROL VALUES ARE GIVEN IN PARENTHESIS

CELLS	HOMOGENATE	SUPERNATANT $(105000g_{av})$	PLASMA MEMBRANE SUBFRACTIONS		
			d 1.12	d 1.14	d 1.16
NORMAL	9.4±0.7 (100)	8.5±0.6 (100)	—	32.1±2.7 (100)	13.5±1.2 (100)
SV$_{40}$ TRANSFORMED: IN VITRO	2.7±0.2 (29)	5.1±0.4 (60)	6.2±0.3	18.1±0.5 (56)	3.1±0.1 (23)
IN VIVO IMPLANT	4.0±0.3 (42)	4.2±0.4 (50)	7.0±0.5	22.1±0.9 (69)	4.0±0.3 (30)

MEANS OF SIX OBSERVATIONS ± S.E.

As for to the methods see Table 5.

Soluble adenylate cyclase.

Table 7 shows the distribution of soluble adenylate cyclase with regard to the total activity of cells.

TABLE 7

Soluble adenylate cyclase activity in cells transformed by oncogenic viruses

SUPERNATANT ($105000g_{av}$) FROM :	% OF TOTAL ACTIVITY
BH FIBROBLASTS TRANSFORMED BY SV40:	
IN VITRO	26
IN VIVO IMPLANT	22
RAUSCHER LEUKEMIC SPLEENS OF BALB/c MICE	18

Data are means of four observations.

Table 8 shows that the soluble adenylate cyclase requires 10 mM theophylline in incubation medium
to inhibit the activity of cyclic AMP PDE. An additional DTE or theophylline is not necessary for enhanced
stability of the enzyme.

TABLE 8

Effect of theophylline on soluble adenylate cyclase
activity in cells transformed by oncogenic viruses

| THEOPHYLLINE mM | SV40 | | RAUSCHER VIRUS |
	IN VITRO	IN VIVO	
0	9	11	6
5	21	25	30
10	32	40	50
20	33	40	53
10 + 10 mM DTE[a]	34	41	52

[a]DTE : DITHIOTHREITOL

As for to the methods see Table 3, with the
exception that the incubation medium contained theophylline and DTE in indicated
concentration.

Results are means of two observations.

The pH dependence of enzyme can be seen in Fig.
4. The optimal common value for investigated transformed cells was pH 8.0.

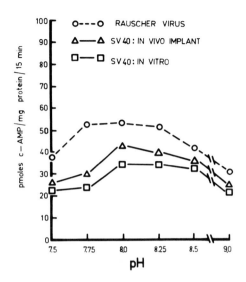

Fig.4. Effect of pH on soluble adenylate cyclase activity in cells transformed by oncogenic viruses.

Results are means of two observations.

The effect of epinephrine, glucagon, PGE_1, $PGF_{2\alpha}$, and fluoride on soluble adenylate cyclase activity is shown in Fig. 5. The enzyme was stimulable by both hormones and fluoride. It is of particular interest that in the Rauscher leukemic spleens of mice it is more than three fold more sensitive to epinephrine than the membrane-bound enzyme. In the same respect the hamster cells transformed by SV 40 show a two fold higher sensitivity to glucagon. The soluble enzyme does not react to prostaglandins.

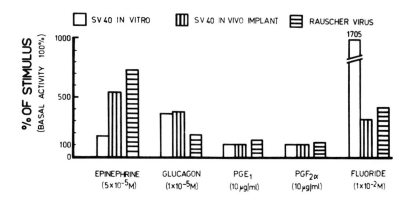

Fig.5. Effect of hormones, prostaglandins, and fluoride on soluble adenylate cyclase activity in cells transformed by oncogenic viruses.
The bars represent means of three observations.

DISCUSSION

When studying the findings referring to the lowered level of cyclic AMP in transformed cells /9., 34./ the following questions may be raised:

a/ can the alterations in cyclic AMP metabolism be brought into connection with the observed changes of cell surface membrane after transformation?

b/ if so, how does the hormone-sensitive adenylate cyclase system and cyclic AMP PDE activities change in the transformed cells, and is this mechanism responsible for decreased cyclic AMP ?

c/ how does the transformed cell try to ensure the cyclic AMP messenger between the cell surface and the nucleus?

Our experimental data do not give adequate answers to all these questions. In some connection, however, they furnish explanation.

Thus it should be underlined that the plasma membranes of cells transformed by DNA and RNA viruses are more differenciated than those of normal ones.

Distribution of hormone-sensitive adenylate cyclase was modified in transformed cells and unidirected independently of transforming agents /DNA or RNA virus/. For this alteration the change of enzyme localizing gene, may be responsible, after transformation. This supposition was confirmed by Eckhart's observation who described the genetic control of plasma membrane using a temperature-sensitive mutant of polyoma virus /ts-3/ as transforming agent. At permissive temperatures which allowed expression of the gene the surface receptors were exposed, whilst at non-permissive temperatures they inactivate the gene and the receptors were covered /35./.

In the plasma membrane subfractions of cells transformed by DNA /SV 40/ and RNA /RLV/ viruses the activity of enzymes synthetizing and decomposing cyclic AMP did not change in a similar manner. In the membrane subfraction the activity of cyclic AMP PDE was considerably higher / expressed in nanomoles/than that of adenylate cyclase /expressed in picomoles/. Activity of the latter enzyme in Rauscher leukemic spleens of mice went together with the increased activity of cyclic AMP PDE, while in SV 40 transformed hamster cells activity of both enzymes decreased. This activity decrease was smaller in the in vivo implant than in the cultured cells. The latter fact calls the attention to the role of a number of regulating factors appearing in vivo, which were also confirmed by the observed sensitivity to prostaglandins in tumor cells growing in vivo.

The fact that the hormonal receptors of adenylate cyclase were transferred to lighter membrane subfraction during transformation means that the transformed cell does not lose its hormonal control. However, in the case of RLV transformed cells the response to epinephrine decreased and at the same time, in contrast to normal cells, a glucagon responsiveness appeared in the lighter subfraction /d 1.12/. A similar abnormal adenylate cyclase response was found in other tumor types. The adenylate cyclase of some pheochromocytomas responded to glucagon, which hormone has no effect on the adenylate cyclase of the normal adrenal medulla /36./.

As we have succeded in demonstrating the epinephrine and glucagon responsiveness separately in membrane subfractions, the existence of discrete epinephrine and glucagon-responsive adenylate cyclase has been confirmed also in investigated transformed cells, as demonstrated previously in liver by Bitensky's group /37.-39./.

The fact that in the transformed cells adenylate cyclase activity was found also in soluble form, may partly mean that this is one indicator of neoplastic state. The physiological role of soluble adenylate cyclase is yet unknown.

Concluding, we have demonstrated evidences of abnormal cyclic AMP metabolism of cells transformed by oncogenic viruses, which can be characterized as follows :

a/ altered distribution of surface membrane subfractions after transformation along sucrose-density gradient ;

b/ altered distribution of adenylate cyclase in these membrane subfractions and a demonstrability of this enzyme also in soluble form in transformed cells ;

c/ decreased activity of adenylate cyclase and changed activity of cyclic AMP PDE in membrane subfractions;

d/ altered responsiveness to hormones of adenylate cyclase ;

e/ hormonal responsiveness of adenylate cyclase transferred to lighter membrane subfractions ;

f/ between the tumor cells growing in vitro and in vivo there are differences in hormonal responsiveness of the adenylate cyclase;

g/ altered hormonal responsiveness of adenylate cyclase depending on transformations either by DNA or RNA viruses.

REFERENCES

/1/ G.A. Robinson, R.W. Butcher and E.W. Sutherland, Cyclic AMP /Acad. Press, New York, 1971/.

/2/ D.F.H. Wallach, in : Current topics in Microbiology and Immunology, 47 /1969/ 152.

/3/ M.Inbar, H. Ben-Bassat and L.Sachs, Nature New Biology, 236 /1972/ 3.

/4/ M.M. Burger, Proc. Nat.Acad.Sci. /USA/, 62 /1969/ 994.

/5/ S. Seki, S.Omura and T.Oda, Gann, 62 /1971/ 89.

/6/ C.V. Perry, G.S. Johnson and I. Pastan, J.Biol. Chem. 246 /1971/ 5785.

/7/ I.Schorr, P. Rathnam, B.B. Saxena and R.L. Ney, J.Biol. Chem. 246 /1971/ 5806.

/8/ D.O. Allen, J.Munshover, H.P. Morris and G. Weber, Cancer Res. 31 /1971/ 557.

/9/ J.R. Sheppard, Nature New Biology, 236 /1972/ 14.

/lo/ P. Emmelot and C.J. Bos, Biochim. Biophys. Acta, 249 /1971/ 285.

/11/ J. F. Perdue, R. Kletzien and K.Miller, Biochim. Biophys. Acta, 249 /1971/ 419.

/12/ R.Sheimin and K. Onodera, Biochim. Biophys.Acta, 274 /1972/ 49.

/13/ P.Emmelot and C.J. Bos, J.Membrane Biol. 9 /1972/ 83.

/14/ J.F. Perdue, R.Kletzien, and V.L. Wray, Biochim. Biophys. Acta, 266 /1972/ 505.

/15/ W.H. Evans, Biochem. J. 116 /1970/ 833.

/16/ M. Barclay, R.K. Barclay, V.P. Skipski, E.S. Essner and O. Terebus-Kekish, Biochim. Biophys. Acta, 255 /1972/931.

/17/ G.S. Johnson and I. Pastan, J.Nat. Cancer Inst. 48 /1972/ 1377.

/18/ P. Chandra and D. Gericke, Naturwissenschaften, 59 /1972/ 205.

/19/ T.K., Ray, Biochim. Biophys.Acta, 196 /197o/1.

/2o/ A.Réthy, A.Trevisani, R.Manservigi and V. Tomasi, submitted for publication.

/21/ V.Tomasi, A.Réthy, and A. Trevisani, Life Sciences, in press /1973/.

/22/ A.B. Sabin and M.A. Koch, Proc. Nat. Acad. Sci. /USA/, 49 /1963/ 304.

/23/ L. Géder, L. Váczi, and E. Jeney, Acta Virologica, 15 /1971/ 35.

/24/ F.D.Tóth, L.Váczi and K. Berencsi, Acta Microbiol. Acad.Sci. /Hungary/ 18 /1971/ 23.

/25/ S.L. Pohl, L. Birnbaumer and M. Rodbell, J.Biol. Chem. 246 /1961/ 1849.

/26/ P. Emmelot and C.J. Bos, Biochim. Biophys. Acta 120 /1966/ 399.

/27/ P.Emmelot, C.J. Bos, E.L. Benedetti and P. Rümke, Biochim. Biophys.Acta, 9o /1964/126.

/28/ S.J. Cooperstein and A. Lazarow, J.Biol. Chem. 189 /1961/ 665.

/29/ W. Mejbaum, Z. Physiol. Chem. 258 /1939/ 117.

/3o/ A. Réthy, V. Tomasi and A. Trevisani, Arch. Biochem. Biophys. 147 /1971/ 36.

/31/ G.V. Marinetti, T.K. Ray and V. Tomasi, Biochem. Biophys. Res. Comm. 36 /1969/ 185.

/32/ A.Réthy, V. Tomasi, A Trevisani and O. Barnabei Biochem. Biophys. Acta, 290 /1972/ 58.

/33/ A.W. Murray, M. Spiszmann and D.E. Atkinson, Science, 171 /1971/ 496.

/34/ J. Otten, G.S. Johnson and I. Pastan, Biochem. Biophys. Res. Comm. 44 /1971/ 1192.

/35/ W. Eckhart, in : The biology of oncogenic viruses, ed. L. Silvestri, /North-Holland, 1971/ p. 68.

/36/ R.N. Dexter and D.D. Allen, Clin. Res. 13/1970/ 601.

/37/ M.W. Bitensky, V. Russel and M. Blanco, Endocrinology, 86 /1970/ 154.

/38/ M.W. Bitensky, V. Russel and W. Robertson, Biochem. Biophys. Res. Comm. 31/1968/ 796.

/39/ R.E. Gorman and M.W. Bitensky, Endocrinology, 87, /1970/ 1075.

ACKNOWLEDGEMENTS

We wish to thank Prof.P.Endes, Institute of Pathology, Medical School of Debrecen, Hungary, for electronmicroscopical examinations. The excellent technical assistance of Miss J.Varga and Mr. Z.Magyari is gratefully acknowledged.

DISCUSSION

G.S. Johnson, National Institutes of Health: I didn't
quite catch, in the case of normal fibroblasts, what
per cent of the total cyclase activity is soluble and also
what per cent is soluble in your SV 40-transformed cells?

A. Réthy, Medical University of Debrecen, Hungary:
As it was demonstrated in Table 4 and Table 7, the normal
fibroblasts contained the soluble adenylate cyclase only
in traces, whilst in the SV 40-transformed fibroblasts
26% and 22% of total activity was soluble depending
on in vitro or in vivo conditions.

G.S. Johnson: How did you homogenize your cells?
What kind of buffer did you use, and what was the
salt in your buffer?

A. Réthy: The homogenization was carried out in
a Dounce homogenizer using bicarbonate buffer 1 mM,
pH 7.5, containing 2 mM Ca^{+2}.

J. Roth, Yale University: I would like to ask a few
questions concerning the method of membrane isolation
that you used. Specifically, do you have any data
on endoplasmic reticulum contamination, such as smooth
endoplasmic reticulum which would contain DPNH-diaphorase
such as described by Wallach in his preparation of
plasma membranes from Ehrlich Ascites carcinoma?
Wallach found that in his initial preparation of plasma
membranes he had not removed a considerable amount
of contamination in the form of smooth E.R. Now if you
express enzyme activity, in this case the activity of
adenyl cyclase, in terms of activity per mg of protein,

the data will be either skewed or obscured by the considerable fraction of protein which is represented by smooth E.R. Also, your data seemed to indicate RNA contamination which would indicate the presence of rough endoplasmic reticulum. Finally, the method does not seem capable of separating smooth E.R. from plasma membrane, at least that fraction of smooth E.R. which sedimented with the plasma membrane until the final step in the Wallach procedure, which is presented in volume eight in *Methods in Enzymology*.

A. Réthy: We have not checked the smooth endoplasmic reticulum contamination, using marker enzymes, in our membrane subfractions. The further characterization of these subfractions is in progress in our laboratory.

PROSTAGLANDINS AND THE ADENYL CYCLASE OF THE CLOUDMAN MELANOMA

J.J. Keirns, P.W. Kreiner, W.A. Brock,
J. Freeman and   M.W.Bitensky
Department of Pathology, Yale University School
of Medicine, New Haven, Connecticut 06510

The adenyl cyclase system occupies a position of central importance in non steriodal hormone biochemistry (1) Understandably there is much interest in how cyclic AMP might function in relation to cancer cell biology. Observations of cyclic AMP effects on the morphology and the biochemistry of transformed cells provide some evidence that cyclic nucleotides can profoundly influence their membrane properties. (2) Cyclic AMP is also known to affect the membrane properties of normal cells producing changes in sodium transport (3), water permeability (4) and hormone release (5). The relationship of cyclic AMP levels to mitotic frequency is also a subject of current interest. While elevated cyclic AMP levels may be associated with diminished mitotic frequency in fibroblasts of skin, (6) elevated cyclic AMP levels appear compatible with increased mitotic frequency in normal adrenal (7), thyroid (8) or ovary (9) and even may be a concomitant of neoplastic transformation when present chronically in ovary (10) and possibly other tissues such as adrenal. Thus general statements implicating elevated or diminished cyclic AMP levels as central etiologic factors in the neoplastic state are really not yet possible. However, the study of cyclase and its related enzyme systems in cancer cells seems of more than pedestrian interest.

Our own interest in the Cloudman mouse melanoma was provoked by the results of studies done with the melanocyte system in the skin of Rana pipiens. We found that cyclic AMP mimics the effects of melanocyte stimulating hormone (MSH) on frog dermal melanocytes (a dispersion of melanosomes especially into the peripheral dendritic processes of the melanocyte) (11). This finding and the fact that methyl xanthines (which inhibit cyclic AMP phosphodiesterase) could darken amphibian skin were taken as partial support for the hypothesis that the regulation of melanocyte metabolism by MSH was mediated by the adenyl cyclase system. Additional support for this idea was provided by Butcher and coworkers in a study which showed that MSH could increase the cyclic AMP content of pigmented dorsal R. pipiens skin while having no effect on the cyclic AMP content of the unpigmented abdominal skin (12). An element still lacking in the proof of the MSH-cyclase hypothesis, was the demonstration that MSH could selectively activate adenyl cyclase in the appropriate broken cell preparations, especially membrane particles derived from homogeneous collections of melanocytes. Initial attempts to pursue this question in amphibian melanocytes were complicated by the mechanical problems associated with preparing membrane fragments from dermal melanocytes (associated with the abundance of collagen) and the fact that the population of dermal melanocytes is loosely dispersed among other cell types, none of which respond to MSH peptides, but most of which contain cyclase molecules exhibiting basal cyclase activity in the absence of added hormones. These difficulties were avoided by doing these experiments on the effect of MSH in broken cells from the Cloudman mouse melanoma, as essentially homogeneous population of mammalian melanocytes which exhibited a vigorous and selective stimulation of adenyl cyclase activity by MSH. Initial studies with this system including the profile of hormonal sensitivity which characterized the cyclase, have been described in detail, (13). The primary features of the systems include responsiveness to both alpha and beta MSH as well as to MSH peptides which have been racemized by brief exposure to tenth normal sodium hydroxide. There is the expected cross reactivity to ACTH, no response to or inhibition by melatonin and minimal activation by catecholamines. The latter observations (with melatonin and norepinephrine) are perhaps contrary to what might have been expected in frog skin (14).

Additional interest in the melanoma from the point of view of the cyclase system and the regulation of gene expression has recently derived from the finding by Pastan (15) that the levels of the enzyme tyrosinase in the melanoma appear to be regulated by cyclic AMP. We have examined both melanotic and relatively amelanotic varieties of the malanoma and in both instances an excellent response to the MSH peptides in broken cell preparations was observed. This suggests that pigment synthesis in the mammalian melanocyte or at least the melanoma melanocyte is regulated by a complex sequence of reactions and that there can be lesions distal to the MSH-cyclase interaction. The relationships of the entire cyclase cascade are especially cogent in assessing any generalizations about the role of cyclic AMP (as an isolated variable) in the biochemistry of cancer cells.

In the present study, we should like to discuss some additional aspects of the regulation and characteristics of the Cloudman melanoma adenyl cyclase system. We will

emphasize the selectivity and efficacy of
prostaglandins as regulators of this cyclase
system in broken cell preparations. The
interaction of calcium with the MSH and
prostaglandin activations of adenyl cyclase, and
the failure of MSH to affect prostaglandin
synthetase activity will be discussed. In this
context we will consider the hypothesis (16)
that prostaglandins are obligatory intermediates
in the activation of any cyclase system by tissue
specific hormones. We will also consider the
distribution of melanoma cyclase in the various
centrifugal fractions derived from homogenates
of melanoma, and finally the effects of various
regulators on the cyclic AMP content of melanoma
slices in which cellular architecture is
relatively preserved. These observations are
briefly discussed in the context of current
understanding of cyclic nucleotide biochemistry
as it might bear on the putative biochemistry of
cancer cells.

MATERIALS AND METHODS

Both the melanotic and relatively amelanotic
strains of the S-91 Cloudman melanoma were
obtained from Dr. Harry Demopoulos of the New
York University School of Medicine. The tumors
were maintained in male mice of the strain DBA/2J
(Jackson Memorial Labs.) and were transplanted
under aseptic conditions by intraperitoneal
injection of finely minced tissue suspended in
0.15M. saline. Tumors grew as encapsulated solid
masses with adhesions to omentum and peritoneum.
The intraperitoneal location produced growth
which was more homogeneous and less necrotic
than the subcutaneous location. Time for
appearance of a 1 cm. tumor was about 2 1/2 weeks.

Tissue was homogenated with a motor driven
Potter-Elvejhem homogenizer (12 strokes, teflon
or glass 4°) in 0.12 M potassium acetate buffer
pH 7.4 which contained 0.03 M KCl. Washed
particles were prepared (from the above

184

homogenates) (13). Tissue slices (0.2mm
thickness) were made with a McElwain chopper
(Ivan Sorvall Co.) at 4°C. Slices were incubated in oxygenated Krebs Ringer bicarbonate for
10 min. at 37°C., and incubations were
terminated by freezing the samples in liquid
nitrogen, grinding with a morter and pestle, and
thawing into 50% acetic acid which contained
[8-3H] cyclic AMP (Schwartz-Mass) to permit
estimation of recovery.

ACTH and MSH were provided by Drs. Lande
and Lerner of Yale University. The
prostaglandins and 7-oxa-13-prostynoic acid were
provided by Drs. Caldwell and Speroff of Yale
University. Indomethacin was a gift from Merke
& Co. Prostaglandins were stored at -20°C. in
absolute ethanol. Immediately before use they
were dried and dissolved in the reaction buffer.
Indomethacin and 7-oxa-13-prostynoic acid were
dissolved in methanol and diluted 1:40 into the
reaction buffer.

Cyclase activity was assayed as previously
described (17). In brief [8-^{14}C] ATP was used
as the substrate. Labeled cyclic AMP with added
cold cyclic AMP for visualization was purified
by descending thin layer chromatography on
polyethyleneimine cellulose for eight hours with
1M ammonium acetate-methanol (2:5). The origin
was then removed by shaving just behind the
cyclic AMP spots, the plates were dried,
rewicked and rechromatographed for 12 hours with
1-butanol-acetic acid-water (2:1:1). Results
were completely reproducible if the chromato-
grams were run at 31°C. The purified cyclic AMP
still on PEI cellulose was shaved directly into
scintillation vials, dispersed by sonication,
and counted with toluene PPO cocktail in the
presence of Cabosil in a Beckman LS 200 liquid
scintillation spectrometer. Assay adenyl cyclase
activity was carried out using a three minute
incubation period at 37°C., in the presence of
1.6mM [8-^{14}C] ATP (45 ci/mole, Schwartz-Mann),

185

5 mM aminophylline, and an ATP regenerating
system (38 mM phosphocreatine and 80 ug/ml
creatine phosphokinase) in buffer 1 (3mM $MgSO_4$,
0.4 mM EDTA, and 32 mM glycylglycine, pH 7.4).
Assay of 3'5' nucleotide phosphodiesterase was
carried out by incubating in the presence of
10^{-4} M [8-$^{-14}$C] cAMP (39 Ci/mole, Schwartz-Mann)
in buffer 1 and measuring the dissappearance of
substrate in 1 min. Protein kinase was assayed
by the method of Kuo and Greengard (18). Protein
concentrations were determined by the method of
Lowry (19). Cyclic AMP levels of tissue slices
were determined by the radioimmunoassay method
of Steiner (20) with minor modifications (21).

Prostaglandin synthetase was assayed by
measuring conversion of labeled arachidonic acid
to labeled prostaglandins [5,6,8,9,11,12,14,15-^{3}
H] arachidonic acid (1,800 Ci/mole, New England
Nuclear) was purified just prior to use by
column chromatography (22). Samples were
incubated in a total volume of 0.1 ml containing
32 mM glycylglycine buffer, pH 7.4 x 10^{-7}M
labeled and 1.6 x 10^{-5}M unlabeled arachidonic
acid, with or without 2 x 10^{-5}M MSH. The
incubation was carried out at 37°C. in a shaking
incubator under air for 20 min. The samples
acidified to pH 2.5 with 1 N HCl, and extracted
twice with 8 mL of ethyl acetate. The combined
ethyl acetate extracts were dried under nitrogen.
Samples were purified by column chromatography
(22) followed by thin layer chromatography (23),
and counted on a Packard Tri-Carb Liquid
Scintillation Counter (Model 3375). Counts were
found both in the E fraction (PGE_2) and in the F
fraction (PGF_2). To further confirm that the
counts in the E fraction were prostaglandin, it
was converted to prostaglandin B (24),
rechromatographed, and the label was found in
the PGB fraction.

RESULTS

The sensitivity of melanoma cyclase to different prostaglandins (PG) is shown in figure 1. Activation by MSH is included for comparison. The magnitude of activation by PGE is 1 1/2 to 2 times greater than that seen with MSH. In the presence of saturating amounts of PGE_1, PGE_2 and PGF_1 MSH produces additional activation of melanoma cyclase. (Table I) MSH activation is also additive with the activation produced by saturating amounts of fluoride (table I). The activation of cyclase by PGE_1 appears to reach saturation at a concentration of 10%/ml. (Figure 2). Activation of cyclase by MSH is lowered by EGTA and restored by calcium. Although fluoride activation is blocked by EGTA this inhibition is not prevented or reversed by calcium or magnesium. PGE_1 activation appears to occur without the calcium dependence found for activation by MSH (table II)

Activation by MSH is partially blocked by 7-0xa-13-prostynoic acid (a prostaglandin antogonist) and by indomethacin (an inhibitor of prostaglandin synthetase) (Fig.3). The concentrations required for both inhibitors, however is quite high and raised questions concerning the specificity and locus of the inhibition. The 30 to 40% inhibition of MSH effects by indomethacin is seen only at concentrations of inhibitor which are 100 times as large as those required for the inhibition of PG synthetase. (table III).

The effects of MSH on PG synthesis were examined in melanoma. The tritiated prostaglandin precursor (arachidonic acid) was readily converted to PGE_2 and PGF_2 by melanoma homogenates. The homogenate produced 2.6 pmoles PGE_2/min/mg protein and 1.0 pmoles PGF_2/min/mg. protein. The rates of synthesis were not influenced by those concentrations of MSH which profoundly activate melanoma cyclase in the same homogenate preparations.

The distribution of cyclase in melanoma homogenates was somewhat atypical in that there was a measurable (15%) amount of total cyclase activity (showing both MSH and PGE_1 responsiveness) in a 200,000 x g supernatent fraction. The bulk of the cyclase activity, however did sediment with the heavy particulate fraction (table IV).

The melanoma homogenates also exhibit phosphodiesterase and protein kinase activities. Both of these cyclase related enzymes appear primarily in the soluble fraction. Phosphodiesterase hydrolyzed 2.6 nmoles of cAMP/ mg protein and showed the usual sensitivity to methyl xanthines. The protein kinase incorporated 7.2 pmole of acid precipitable PO_4 into histone/min/mg protein in response to 10^{-5}Molar cAMP. The K 1/2 for cAMP was about 10^{-7}Molar. Cyclic AMP sensitivity was markedly enhanced by preincubation of homogenates at 30° for 20 min.

The melanoma cyclase was also evaluated as a slice preparation. Basal levels of cyclic AMP (.23 pmole/mg of tissue) were markedly increased by MSH (.51 pmoles) and PGE_1 (0.84 pmoles). Attempts were made to detect ectopic receptors with parathormone, vasopressin, glucagon, TSH, and FSH. The melanoma slices showed hormone sensitivity which was confined to PGE_1 MSH and related (ACTH) peptides. Half maximal activation of melanoma homogenate cyclase is seen at $5x10^{-7}$ M MSH. The slice preparation showed half maximal activation at 2×10^{-7}M MSH, a concentration somewhat higher than would be expected to function in vivo.

DISCUSSION

Regulation of the adenyl cyclase system in the mouse Cloudman melanoma is quite complex, and appears to involve prostaglandins and calcium as well as MSH. The cyclase of the melanoma shows a marked and selective response to PGE_1 even in broken cell preparations. This magnitude of PGE_1 activation of melanoma cyclase in membrane fragments has not been observed in other tissues. The stimulation of cyclase by PGE_1 is significantly greater than the stimulation produced by porcine MSH. Since the amino acid sequence of mouse MSH is not known it is conceivable,though unlikely, that this apparent greater efficacy of PGE_1 rests in the preference of the tissue for mouse rather than pig MSH. Such a preference for mouse MSH could not be the result of greater binding affinity since both the prostaglandins and the peptides are being used at the saturating concentrations. Further, there is no species variation for all of the αMSH peptides (5 species) which have thus far been sequenced. It seems rather that the potential for activation is greater for the prostaglandins than for the peptides, and that prostaglandins are important regulators of the melanoma cyclase.

We emphasize that when melanocyte peptides are used in combination with the prostaglandins they provide additional stimulation of cyclase. This additivity coupled with the fact that MSH has no effect on prostaglandin synthetase suggests that prostaglandins are not obligatory intermediates in the cyclase activation sequence. Further, while indomethacin which is a known inhibitor of prostaglandin synthetase (25) does in fact inhibit the activation of melanoma cyclase by MSH, it does so at concentrations 100 times greater than those required to inhibit prostaglandin synthetase. Hence, the inhibitor may act at the hormone receptor or some other locus and have little, if anything, to do with prostaglandin synthesis in the homogenate or

washed particle preparations in which cyclase is
being assayed. On the other hand activation by
MSH as well as PGE_1 is antagonized in a seemingly
competitive manner by 7-oxa-13-prostynoic acid
and our data do not exclude the possibility that
the hormone (MSH) promotes release of sequestered
endogenous prostaglandins.

The requirement for calcium in the
activation of melanoma cyclase by MSH is
analogous to the calcium requirement for
activation of adrenal cortical cyclase by ACTH.
(26). The lack of a calcium requirement in the
activation of melanoma cyclase by prostaglandins
suggest that MSH and prostaglandins insert into
the cyclase activation sequence at different
points. Certainly the profound structural
dissimilarities between the two classes of
activators is compatible with the concept that
they possess independent binding sites for
activation of cyclase.

The presence of a cyclic AMP activated
protein kinase in the melanoma is not surprising,
since such an enzyme has been demonstrated or
implicated as a member of the sequence by which
cyclic AMP promotes the elaboration of hormone
directed specialized cell functions in many
tissues. Melanoma protein kinase may mediate
the cyclic AMP directed induction of tyrosinase,
the thus participate in the regulation of pigment
synthesis. The fact that in at least some
amelanotic melanomas the cyclase system is intact
up to and including the protein kinase, suggests
that the lesion in melanin synthesis in such
tumors is probably distal to the protein kinase.

The levels of cyclase and cyclic AMP in the
melanoma would appear not to be deminished as
judged by a variety of criteria. Direct
measurements of basal and hormone stimulated
levels of cyclic AMP in slice preparations are
greater than the levels found in normal liver,
and the amounts are more than adequate for

activation of the protein kinase. Other evidence for excellent cyclic AMP production is the dense pigmentation of the tumor produced by vigorous melanin synthesis. The normal pigmentation of the host animals argues that there is an adequate supply of MSH for both tumor and epidermal receptors.

In spite of the neoplastic characteristics of the melanoma (as exemplified by increased mitotic frequency, abnormal morphology with rounding of the cells with the loss of their processes, distal metasteses, and invasion of contiguous structures,) a large fraction of the cyclase regulatory apparatus appears entirely intact (in much the same way as we previously found for a variety of Morris hepatomas (27)). These findings imply that a deficiency in the adenyl cyclase system cannot be unequivocally assigned as a primary locus of abnormality in the development of the neoplastic state in the Cloudman melanoma.

ACKNOWLEDGEMENTS

This work was supported by USPHS grants 1-R01-AM-15016 and 1-R01-CA-1344. J.J. Keirns is a fellow of the Jane Coffin Childs Memorial Fund for Medical Research.

REFERENCES

1. I. Pastan, Sci.Amer., Sept. 1972, p. 97
   M.W. Bitensky and R.E. Gorman, Ann.Rev.Med.
   23 (1972) 263.
2. A.W. Hsie, C.Jones and T.T. Puck, Proc.Nat.
   Acad.Sci. USA 68 (1971) 1648.
   G.S. Johnson, R.W. Friedman and I Pastan,
   Proc.Nat.Acad.Sci. USA (1971) 425.
3. J.Orloff and J.S. Handler, J.Clin.Invest. 41
   (1962) 702.
4. J. Orloff and J.S. Handler, Amer.J.Med. 42
   (1967) 757.
5. M.W. Bitensky and R.E. Gorman, Prog.Biophys.
   Mol.Biol. (1972) in press.
6. J.J. Voorhees, and E.A. Duell, Arch.Derm.104
   (1971) 352.
7. D.G. Grahame-Smith, R.W. Butcher, R.L. Ney
   and E.W. Sutherland, J.Biol.Chem. 242 (1967)
   5535.
8. L.M. Klainer, Y.M. Chi, S.L. Freidberg, T.W.
   Rall and E.W. Sutherland, J.Biol.Chem. 237
   (1962) 1239.
9. F. Murad, B.S. Strauch, and M. Vaughan
   Biochim.Biophys.Acta 177 (1969) 591.
10. W.U. Gardner, J.Nat.Can.Inst. 26 (1961) 829.
11. M.W. Bitensky, and S.R. Burstein, Nature, 208
    (1965) 1282.
12. K.Abe, R.W. Butcher, W.E. Nicholson, W.E.
    Burd, R.A. Liddle and G.W. Liddle
    Endocrinology 84 (1969) 362.
13. M.W. Bitensky, H.B. Demopoulos and V. Russell
    in pigmentation:Its Genesis and Biologic
    Control, ed.V. Riley (Appleton-Century-Croft
    New York, 1972) p. 247.
14. A.B. Lerner, Nature, 184 (1959) 674.
15. G.S. Johnson and I. Pastan, Nature New
    Biology 237 (1972) 269.
16. F.A. Kuehl, Jr. J.L. Humes, J. Tarnoff, V.J.
    Cirillo, and E.A. Ham, Science, 169 (1970)
    883.

17. A.M. Spiegal and M.W. Bitensky,
    Endocrinology 85 (1969) 638.
18. J.F. Kuo and P. Greengard, J.Biol.Chem. 245
    (1970) 2493.
19. O.H. Lowry, N.O. Rosebrough and A.L. Randall
    J.Biol.Chem 193 (1951) 265.
20. A.L. Steiner, D.M. Kipnis, R. Utiger and
    C. Parker, Proc.Nat.Acad.Sci. USA 64 (1969)
    367.
21. R.C. Wagner, P. Kreiner, R.J. Barrnett and
    M.W. Bitensky, Proc.Nat.Acad.Sci.USA 69
    (1972) 3175.
22. B.W. Caldwell, S. Burstein, W.A. Brock and
    L.Speroff, J.Clin.Endo.Met. 33 (1971) 171.
23. K. Green and B. Samuelson, J.Lipid Res. 5
    (1964) 117.
24. R.M. Zusman, Prostaglandins 1 (1972) 167.
25. J.R. Vane, Nature New Biology 231 (1971) 232
26. R.J. Lefkowitz, J.Roth and I Pastan 228
    (1970) 864.
27. R.E. Gorman and M.W. Bitensky, Philadelphia
    Hepatoma Conf. 1971.

TABLE I

ADDITIVE EFFECTS OF MSH, PROSTAGLANDINS AND FLUORIDE

ADENYL CYCLASE ACTIVITY

Regulator	Without MSH	With MSH
Control	1.7	5.9
MSH	5.9	5.9
PGE_1	8.5	11.0
PGE_2	2.6	6.8
PGF_1	2.3	6.5
Fluoride	7.5	10.0

Activities are expressed as nmoles cAMP/10 min./ mg. of protein. Regulator concentrations are as follows: MSH 50 μg/ml., PGE_1, PGE_2, and PGF_1 10 μg/ml, and fluoride 10mM. Experiments were carried out with whole homogenate preparations.

TABLE II

ROLE OF CALCIUM IN MELANOMA CYCLASE ACTIVITION

	Control	MSH	E_1	Fluoride
Control	2.0	5.5	8.0	4.5
EGTA	1.7	3.7	7.9	2.5
EGTA+Ca^{++}	2.0	6.0	7.8	2.3
EGTA+Mg^{++}	1.8	4.0	8.3	2.9

Activities are expressed as a nmole cAMP/10 min./ mg. of protein. Reagent concentrations are as follows: MSH 50γ/ml., PGE_1 10γ/ml., fluoride 10mM, EGTA 7mM, Ca^{++} and Mg^{++} 1mM. Whole homogenate preparations were used throughout.

TABLE III

INHIBITION OF CYCLASE ACTIVATION BY INDOMETHACIN

MSH Concentrations (γ/ml.) $\longrightarrow$	0	6.25	12.5	2 5
Indomethacin (50γ/ml.)	(Adenyl Cyclase Activity)			
Indomethacin (50γ/ml.)	0.7	0.9	1.0	1.2
Indomethacin (5γ/ml.)	1.2	1.4	2.1	2.9
Control	1.2	1.5	2.1	3.0

Activities are expressed as nmole cAMP/10 min./ mg. of protein. Whole homogenate preparations were used throughout.

TABLE IV

SEDIMENTATION CHARACTERISTICS OF CYCLASE SYSTEM IN MELANOMA HOMOGENATES

Tissue (g) sedimented	Time of centri- fugation	Basal Activity	MSH-Stimulated	PGE$_1$-Stimulated
1,000	1/2 hr.	1.5 (33%)	3/1 (46%)	6.5 (54%)
10,000	1/2 hr.	0.9 (20%)	1.0 (15%)	2.3 (19%)
50,000	1 hr.	0.7 (16%)	0.5 (7%)	1.4 (12%)
200,000	1 hr.	0.5 (11%)	0.5 (7%)	0.7 (6%)
200,000 Supernatent	1 hr.	0.9 (20%)	1.7 (25%)	1.1 (9%)
Total		4.5 (100%)	6.8 (100%)	12/1 (100%)

Specific activities are expressed as nmoles/10 min./mg. of protein.
Number in parenthesis is the percent of total basal, hormone or PGE$_1$
stimulated activity. Sedimented particulate fractions were suspended in
an equal volume of reaction buffer. [MSH] was 50 ɤ/ml. and [PGE$_1$] was
10 ɤ/ml.

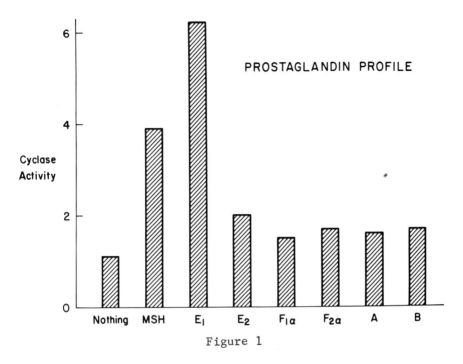

PROSTAGLANDIN PROFILE

Figure 1

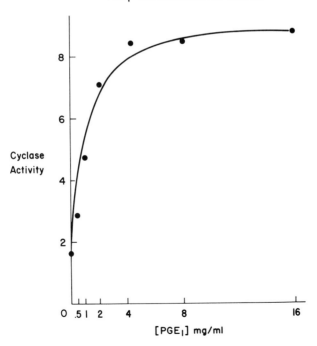

PGE₁ CONCENTRATION CURVE

Figure 2

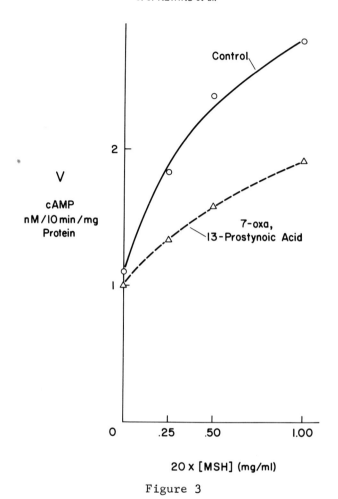

Figure 3

DISCUSSION

G.S. Johnson, National Institutes of Health: It's interesting that in the Cloudman melanoma S 91 cell line, which we grew in culture, was completely unresponsive to prostaglandin. We did not test MSH, but the dibutyryl cyclic AMP did cause considerable pigment production. I was wondering if you'd have any comments on this, considering the possibility that prostaglandins could be merely activating a contaminating adenylate cyclase in your melanoma.

M. Bitensky, Yale University: I think that the only way to answer this question will be to do the obvious studies in the tissue culture system with the hormones and with the prostaglandins. There are differences. The melanomas evolve, with respect to their generation time, the time required to reach something like 2 or 1 centimeter. Ours now are growing for about $2\frac{1}{2}$ weeks to reach that size. I think that the possibility that a large part of the prostaglandin response is contributed by the endothelial contaminants is a very strong one. I rather suspect, however, that the melanoma may also have an E_1 response. There are, as you know, many deletions in hormone sensitivities in going from solid tumors to tissue culture. Whether these can all be explained in terms of our endothelial cell findings or whether there are true changes remains to be seen. For instance, in some of the hepatoma tissue cultures where the solid tumors exhibit very lovely epinephrin and glucagon responses in culture, one or the other are lost. I should add that the endothelial cells from the fat pad exhibit a very nice glucagon sensitivity, and the melanoma does not.

I. Pastan, National Institutes of Health: Let me add one comment to that please. There are other cell types also present. One of these, of course, is the fibroblast, which is prostaglandin responsive.

M. Bitensky: In looking at EM's of these tumors, the reticular endothelium elements and fibroblast elements are surprisingly sparse. I think that the contribution made by fibroblasts in this tissue is really minimal, not to belittle their very excellent prostaglandin response. I think that's not what we're seeing. I would vote either for the endothelial contaminant or the hepatoma itself.

R. A. Hickie, University of Saskatchewan: When you speak about phosphodiesterase, are you talking about the cyclic AMP phosphodiesterase?

M. Bitensky: Yes.

R.A. Hickie: And you mentioned that it's distributed mainly in the supernatant?

M. Bitnesky: Yes.

R.A. Hickie: Have you determined whether any is particulate-bound?

M. Bitensky: A very small fraction is found in the particulate-fraction. I would say it varies from preparation to preparation, but never exceeds 10%.

R.A. Hickie: Have you tried the effects of prostaglandin E_1 on liver?

M. Bitensky: Yes. Prostaglandin E_1 is a very good activator of hepatic cyclase in washed membranes in crude washed membranes, and in whole homogenate. You can get a very nice response with E_1 at 5 gamma/ml.

R.A. Hickie: I haven't been successful in getting liver adenyl cyclase activation with PG_1, and from the literature, there seems to be some discrepancy as to whether or not PGE_1 actually activates adenyl cyclase.

M. Bitensky: I'm confused now in my recollection of which, we work with six of them, E_1, E_2, F_{1a}, F_{2a}, A, and B. I remember one of them producing a really nice response which was in between the fluoride and glucagon response in magnitude. I'll be dogmatic and say that there's a good prostaglandin response, but now you've made me question whether it's E_1 or not.

Klein, N.Y. University: You demonstrated that in your particles in washed membranes, that there was a specificity for prostaglandin response and it was E_1 giving the most activation. Did this hold up in your non-readily sedimentable fraction, although the activity of the cyclase was small in those fractions? Wasn't there also specificity?

M. Bitensky: That's a good question and we haven't done those experiments to see. The experiments which were done to rank the activity of the prostaglandins were done primarily in washed particles, and the distribution and different centrifugal cuts just used E_1. We haven't repeated that type of profile in the soluble fraction and I think it would be interesting to look.

H.H. Tai, New York University Medical Center: I have two questions. The first one is concerned with your whole cell preparations. I wonder if you have tried the experiment to see whether addition of some prostaglandin synthetase inhibitors, such as indomethacin or meclofenamate, to your preparations has any effect on the elevation of cyclic AMP induced by MSH.

M. Bitensky: It's a very nice experiment. We have not tried that. I do know, however, that the indomethacin

inhibition of other cell cyclase systems, specifically,
thyroid and ovary, have been done in intact cell preparations.
I think all of these experiments are somewhat marred
by the very high concentrations of indomethacin needed,
even in the intact cell, and the concentrations have invariably
been much higher than the concentrations required to
block prostaglandin synthetase.

H.H. Tai: The second question is concerned with
your broken cell preparations. Have you treated your
preparation with prostaglandin dehydrogenase, a prostaglandin
inactivating enzyme, and any effect on the MSH stimulated
cyclic AMP formation the adenyl cyclase system?

M. Bitensky: That's another good experiment that
we haven't done.

L. Mandel, Merck Institute: Have you measured
prostaglandin levels in the melanoma in the presence
and absence of MSH?

M. Bitensky: We haven't done the native levels
because the sensitivity of our immuno assay and our antibody
binding characteristics are not all that we would like
them to be. We have just done the ability of the tissue
to convert tritiated arachidonic acid to various prostaglandins
in the presence and absence of MSH. In other words,
we've done the cyclase assay and not the cyclic AMP content
assay in extrapolation. I think that those experiments
will be very useful.

L. Mandel: Couldn't the additivity between MSH
and PGE be explained on the basis of multiple cell types
in your system?

M. Bitensky: Well, this is always true, and I agree.
I think that the additivity that we found in liver was,
in my mind, convincingly attributed to the paracide itself.
I think that the additivity here will ultimately depend

on doing this in a tissue culture system where responsiveness
to all of the activators is preserved, but I think this is
a good criticism.

I. Pastan: May I continue that line for a moment
and ask if anyone has measured prostaglandin levels
in cells after stimulation by a polypeptide hormone?

L. Mandel: Well, Dr. Kuehl's group in the Merck
Institute has been looking at changes in prostaglandin
levels in the presence and absence of leutinizing hormone
in mouse ovaries. There are no changes in prostaglandins
due to LH. On the other hand, in long-term incubations
for up to 3 hours, one can see changes in prostaglandin
levels due to LH. In addition, we have found that dibutyryl
cyclic AMP itself under certain circumstances can raise
prostaglandin F levels.

I. Pastan: I would like to make two comments about
those experiments. In the intact ovary, there are capillaries,
also, the rate of rise of the prostaglandins is retarded
and occurs much more slowly than the rate of rise of
cyclic AMP in response to LH.

L. Mandel: To answer Dr. Pastan's question in
another light, I think that Burke has measured changes
in prostaglandin in cultured thyroid cells in the presence
and absence of TSH, and I think he's shown elevations.

C. Dalton, Hoffman-La Roche: In your schematic
diagram, you showed the presence of GTP. GTP has
been shown to be an activator of the adenyl cyclase
in membrane preparations. Do you, in fact, have any
data from your homogenate preparations?

M. Bitensky: We have some preliminary data on
this: it looks like GTP appears to help activation by
MSH but I can't really say that it's absolutely indispensable,
but there's a caveat about during these experiments

and that is that in Rodbel's experiments, and those of
others showing GTP activation are done on extensively
purified membranes. One of the benefits of the extensive
purification is to remove endogenous guanine nucleotides.
If these are not removed, and if you try the experiments
in cruder preparations, you're never going to see a
GTP activation. One of the criteria that will help to
understand whether one has gotten the membranes in
the right condition, is that they're almost not responding
to hormone at all. Under those conditions one can see
some stimulation with GTP. This has been done for a
variety of tissues. There's also a report, and I don't
remember the details, that the activation of some cyclases
by prostaglandins appears to be assisted by GTP.

G. Krishna, National Institutes of Health: Should
the homogenate include platelets, you can get an effect
of GTP. That means there is some kind of contamination
of GTP there so that you can get an effect of prostaglandin;
but over and above it, you can get a GTP effect in purified
membranes, again depending on the GTP concentration
and other aspects. It is absolutely essential that you
need GTP for the prostaglandin effect.

H. Sheppard, Hoffman-La Roche: I have just one
comment and a question. As far as the GTP effect is concerned,
we've also seen it with erythrocyte ghosts from freshly
prepared hemolysates. The GTP is a potent enhancer
and protector of catecholamine stimulation of the adenylate
cyclase. I would like to ask a question about the inhibitory
effects of indomethacin. Did you notice any affect on
phosphodiesterase?

M. Bitensky: I haven't looked at the affects of indomethecin on phosphodiesterase. Under the conditions
of our experiments, we've had something like 7.7×10^{-3}
M of aminophylline in the reaction mix. Are you aware
of phosphodiesterase activation by indomethecin?

H. Sheppard: No, I'm aware of an inhibition, not with that particular tissue, but with some other tissues.

I. Pastan: I would like to make one last comment. Dr. Bitensky raised the issue concerning the role of cyclic AMP in controlling the growth rate of all types of tumors. Most of the discussions yesterday referred to the fact that cyclic AMP seems to control the growth rate of transformed embryo cells or fibroblasts, and there's no reason necessarily to believe, and I would not like people to leave here believing, that cyclic AMP does this in all kinds of tumors. I think it is unclear whether it has a regulatory role in other kinds of tumors.

M. Bitensky: That was the intent of my remark. I would feel very much the same way. I think that if one looks at a number of normal tissues, whether this represents a different enzymatic armamentarium or what, cyclic AMP can either increase or decrease mitotic frequency. There is one group of experiments which were done by Gardner quite a while back, where ovaries were placed in spleens and in this environment, the estrogen produced is conjugated immediately by passage through the hepatic portal system. This type of ovary is chronically exposed to elevated gonadotropins and very often becomes carcinomatous. Although at the time these experiments were done, the levels of cyclic AMP were not measured, I think there's enough data to say that it's reasonable to conclude that in the presence of elevated gonadotrophins, the levels of cyclic AMP in the ovary are elevated so that one can even point to conditions where increase levels of cyclic AMP are associated with neoplastic transformation. I think, however, although I have no data, and no right to comment on the transformed cell studies which are very elegant and very exciting, that the collection of cell membrane characteristics which can be influenced by cyclic AMP is startling and striking, and it is not unreasonable to inquire whether these phenomena will be observed in a variety of tumors.

ROLE OF CYCLIC AMP IN THE DIFFERENTIATION OF NEUROBLASTOMA CELL CULTURE

Kedar N. Prasad
Department of Radiology, University of Colorado Medical
Center, Denver, Colorado

Many studies now indicate that cyclic AMP reversibly affects the growth and morphology of several mammalian non-
nerve cells in culture (1 - 5). This paper reviews our
previous studies and presents some new data to show that
cyclic AMP may be involved in irreversible "differentiation" of mouse neuroblastoma cells in culture. The "differentiated" cells for the most part resemble mature neurons. A few non-cyclic AMP agents can produce some of the
changes that are produced by cyclic AMP without changing
the intracellular level of cyclic AMP.

Some Features of Neuroblastoma Cells
The procedures for culturing and maintenance of mouse
neuroblastoma cells were previously described (6). Neuroblastoma cells have a relatively high rate of glycolysis
(7) and contain some features of differentiated neurons
such as tyrosine hydroxylase (8), choline acetyltransferase
(8), acetylcholinesterase (8) and catechol-o-methyltrans-
ferase (9), but lacks tryptophan hydroxylase (10, 11).

Isolation of Clones having different Neuronal Properties
We have isolated four types of neuroblastoma clones (10)
representing four neuronal cell types (Table 1). These include: (a) clone with tyrosine hydroxylase (TH), but no
choline acetyltransferase (ChA), (b) clone with ChA but no
TH, (c) clone with neither TH nor ChA and (d) clone with
both TH and ChA. Amano et. al. (11) were first to isolate
the first three types of clones. Tryptophan hydroxylase
activity was not demonstrable even after treatment with dibutyryl cyclic AMP. The absence of enzyme for serotonin
synthesis indicates that neuroblastoma cells during malignant transformation may become like neural crest cells
which also give rise to at least three primary neurons,
acetylcholine synthesizing neurons, catecholamine synthesizing neurons and sensory neurons which synthesize neither
of the compounds.
The next obvious question arose whether or not human

Table 1. Basal Level of Neural Enzymes in Various
Neuroblastoma Clones

Clones	Tyrosine Hydroxylase (Pmol Product/30 min /10^6 cells)	Choline Acetyl-transferase (Pmol Product/15 min/ 10^6 cells)	Acetylcholinesterase (Pmol AcTc hydro-lysed/min 10^6 cells)
NBA$_2$(1)	0.6 ± 0.1*	0.0	2800 ± 600
NBP$_2$	15.1 ± 0.3	166 ± 39	2400 ± 290
NBDB⁻	0.0	0.0	1400 ± 120
NBE⁻	0.0	266 ± 74	3100 ± 500
L-cells	0.0	0.0	2000 ± 310
Brain	600[1]	1500[1]	5670[2]

*Standard deviation

[1] Mouse caudate nucleus per/mg tissue (J. C. Waymire, Personal communication.)

[2] Rat cortex homogenate per/mg tissue (F. Hobbiger and R. Lancaster, J. Neurochem. 18, 1741-1749 (1971).

The data has been summarized from a previous publication (10).

neuroblastoma tumors which are presumed to have only adrenergic cells, have more than one neuronal cell type. Indeed, we have demonstrated (Table 2) the presence of cholinergic cells in human ganglioneuroma and neuroblastoma
tumors (12).

Cells of all clones grow with a doubling time of about
18 - 24 hours, show spontaneous morphological differentiation varying from 1 to 15 percent and produce tumors when
injected subcutaneously into A/J mice.

Cyclic AMP and Morphological "Differentiation"

Dibutyryl- and monobutyryl- derivatives of cyclic AMP
which penetrate cells probably more easily and are less
susceptible to cyclic AMP phosphodiesterase (PDE) (13) were
used to investigate the role of cyclic AMP in the differentiation of neuroblastoma cells in culture. Prostaglandin
(PG_1) increases the intracellular level of cyclic AMP by
stimulating adenylate cyclase (14). Theophylline, 4-(3-bu-
toxy-4-methoxybenzyl)-2-imidazolidinone (RO20-1724), 4-(3-
dimethoxybenzyl)-2-imidazolidinone (RO7-2956), and papaverine increase the cyclic AMP level by inhibiting the PDE
activity (15, 16). Therefore, in order to show further the
involvement of cyclic AMP in the differentiation of neuroblastoma cells, the above PDE inhibitors were used. Recently ICN Nucleic Acid Research Institute of California
has synthesized several 8-substituted analogs of cyclic
AMP. We have used many of them in the present study. The
procedures for making solutions of all agents were previously described (17 - 20).

Analogs of cyclic AMP (17, 20, 21), prostaglandin E_1
(18) and PDE inhibitors (19) caused morphological "differentiation" of neuroblastoma cells as shown by the formation of axons-like processes and enlargement of nucleus and
soma (Figure 1A-D). Some cells which did not form axons-
like processes also increased in size. Table 3 shows the
relative potency of various agents in causing morphological
"differentiation". PGE_1, PDE inhibitors and 8-benzylthio
cyclic AMP were more effective than dibutyryl cyclic AMP.
No significant cell death occurred after the above treatments and the viability of attached cells as determined by
the uptake of supravital stain (trypan blue in 1 percent
saline) was similar to that of control cells (90 - 95%).

PGE_1 and RO20-1724 increased the cyclic AMP level by
four-fold (40 pmol/mg protein) 3 days after treatment. On

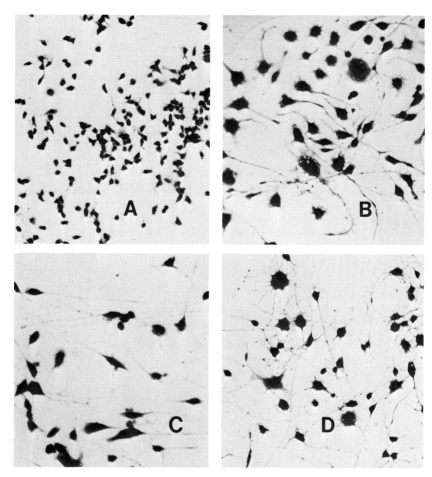

Figure 1. Neuroblastoma cells (50,000) were plated in the
Falcon plastic dishes and dibutyryl cyclic AMP (0.5 mM),
prostaglandin (PG)E$_1$ (10 µg/ml) and 4-(3-butoxy-4-methoxy-
benzyl)-2-imidazolidinone (RO20-1724, 200 µg/ml) were added
separately 24 hours later. The cells were fixed in diluted
formaldehyde (1:10 in distilled water) for 30 seconds,
rinsed quickly and then stained with 1 percent cresyl vio-
let for 2 min. Cells were air dried and oil immersion was
added before taking photomicrographs. Control cells (A)
showed small round cells growing in clumps (5 days after
plating). Dibutyryl cyclic AMP (B) PGE$_1$ (C) and RO20-1724
(D) treated cells (5 days after plating). Original Mag. x
80 (17 - 19) .

Table 2. Choline Acetyltransferase Level in Human
Neuroblastoma and Ganglioneuroma

Type of Tumor	Treatment	Choline Acetyltransferase Activity (pmol/15 min/mg protein)
Human Neuroblastoma Culture	Control	1820 ± 246*
Bone marrow of Human Neuroblastoma	Homogenized	360 ± 20
Human Ganglioneuroma Tissue	Homogenized	180 ± 20
Bone marrow of normal subject	Homogenized	0
Mouse L-cell Culture	Control	0
Mouse Caudate Nucleus	Homogenized	1500**

*Standard deviation

**Per mg of tissue (J. C. Waymire, (unpublished observation)

Data has been taken from a previous publication (12).

removal of the drug 3 days after treatment, the cyclic AMP
level remained high. Another study (22) also shows that
PGE$_1$ increases cyclic AMP level in other neuroblastoma
clone. These data indicate that the morphological differentiation of neuroblastoma cells appears to be linked with a
high intracellular level of cyclic AMP.

The number of morphologically differentiated cells after
PGE$_1$-treatment was time and concentration dependent (18).
A significant increase in the number of differentiated
cells occurred 24 hours after treatment (Figure 2); but
cell division did not stop until the 3rd day (Figure 3).
This indicates that the inhibition of cell division may be
secondary to the induction of morphological differentiation.
The kinetics of morphological differentiation and growth
after treatment with dibutyryl cyclic AMP or PDE inhibitors
(17, 19) were similar to those after PGE$_1$-treatment.

3',5' cyclic AMP, 5' AMP, theophylline, some 8-substitu-
ted analogs of cyclic AMP (8-hydroxyethyl thio-, 8-amino-,
8-hydroxyethylamino and 8-methylamino cyclic AMP), adenosine triphosphate and adenosine diphosphate inhibited cell
growth without causing morphological differentiation. Theophylline, a well known inhibitor of PDE did not increase
cyclic AMP level. These data indicate that the inhibition
of cell division is not sufficient for the expression of
morphological differentiation.

Like cyclic AMP, guanosine 3',5' cyclic monophosphate
(cyclic GMP) is also present in mammalian cells (23).
Therefore, the effects of cyclic GMP on neuroblastoma cell
culture were examined. Neither cyclic GMP, nor N^2-2'-0-di-
butyryl cyclic GMP caused morphological differentiation,
although both agents inhibited cell division.

Irreversability of Growth Inhibition and Morphological Differentiation

The morphological differentiation and inhibition of
growth induced by dibutyryl cyclic AMP, PGE$_1$ or RO20-1724
for the most part were irreversible (Figure 3) provided the
drug was present in the medium for at least 3 - 4 days (17
- 19). This is in contrast to the observation made on non-
nerve cells in which cyclic AMP-effects are reversible at
all times soon after the removal of the drug (3 - 5).

Requirements for the Expression of Differentiated Phenotype

Vinblastine sulfate and cytochalasin B which interfere

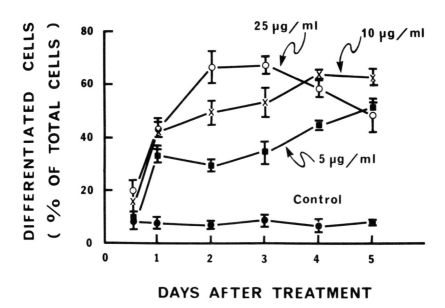

Figure 2. Formation of morphological differentiated cells as a function of time and prostaglandin (PG)E$_1$ concentration. Cells (50,000) were plated in Falcon plastic dishes (60 mm) and various concentrations of PGE$_1$ were added 24 hours later. A total of 300 - 500 cells were counted and the number of morphologically differentiated cells was expressed as the percentage of total cells. Each value represented an average of 8 samples. Bars at point were standard deviations (18) .

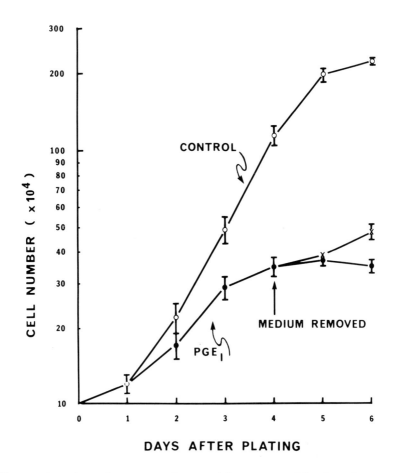

Figure 3. Growth curve of neuroblastoma cells in vitro. Cells were plated in Falcon plastic dishes (60 mm) and Prostaglandin E_1 (10 µg/ml) was added 24 hours later. Prostaglandin E_1 was removed from one group of dishes and fresh growth medium was added 3 days later. In another group of dishes fresh growth medium containing 10 µg/ml of PGE_1 was replaced at the same time. The growth medium in control dishes was also changed. The cell number was counted in a Coulter counter. Each point represented an average of five or six samples. Bars at each point were standard deviations (18).

Table 3. Effect of Various Cyclic AMP Agents on the
Neuroblastoma Cells in Culture

Treatment	Differentiated Cells (% of total cells)
Control	9.0 ± 2.0*
Monobutyryl cyclic AMP (0.5 mM)	47 ± 5.0
Dibutyryl Cyclic AMP (0.5 mM)	51.0 ± 4.8
Prostaglandin E_1 (10 µg/ml)	72.0 ± 5.0
Prostaglandin E_2 (10 µg/ml)	70.0 ± 4.2
RO20-1724 (200 µg/ml)	71.0 ± 5.4
RO7-2956 (200 µg/ml)	54.0 ± 4.7
Papaverine (25 µg/ml)	79.0 ± 2.5
8-benzylthio cyclic AMP (400 µg/ml)	66.0 ± 4.5
8-thio cyclic AMP (200 µg/ml)	30 ± 3.0

For quantitating the number of differentiated cells, cells
(50,000) were plated in plastic dishes and treated with
drug 24 hours after plating. The cells with cytoplasmic
processes greater than 50 µm in length were considered morphologically differentiated. At least 300 cells were
counted and the number of differentiated cells were expressed as percent of total cells. Each value represents
an average of 6 - 8 samples. The data were taken from previous publications (17 - 19).

*Standard deviation

with the assembly of microtubules and microfilaments, respectively, completely blocked the axon formation induced
by dibutyryl cyclic AMP, PGE$_1$, inhibitors of PDE and 8-ben-
zylthio cyclic AMP. Cyloheximide, an inhibitor of protein
synthesis, completely inhibited axon formation, whereas
actinomycin D, an inhibitor of RNA synthesis did not. Thus
the expression of differentiated phenotype requires at
least the assembly of microtubules and microfilaments and
the synthesis of new protein (24), but no RNA synthesis.
The inhibitors used in this study are known to affect several other cellular parameters; in addition to those which
are mentioned here. Therefore, the above conclusion regarding the requirements for the expression of differentiated phenotype should be considered incomplete.

Sensitivity of Neuroblastoma Clones to Cyclic AMP

Cells of all neuronal cell types are sensitive to cyclic
AMP in causing morphological differentiation, however, some
clones irrespective of their neuronal cell type are sensitive to PGE$_1$ but not to RO20-1724 (inhibitor of PDE) and
vice versa (10, 20).

Tumorgenicity of Differentiated Cells

Control cells when injected subcutaneously produced tumors in all animals, whereas the tumorgenecity of differentiated cells (4 days after treatment) was partially or completely abolished (25). The uncloned cells was used as it is
more pertinent to in vivo condition. Since some cells were
responsive to PGE$_1$ but not to PDE inhibitor and vice versa,
PGE$_1$ was combined with RO20-1724 to produce a maximal effect on differentiation. Indeed, cells treated as above
did not produce tumors (Table 4). The above agents had no
effect on the growth of neuroblastoma cells in vivo. This
may be due to the fact that doses of drugs which might have
produced differentiation are toxic for the animals.

Comparative study between Control and "Differentiated" Cells

Several studies were performed in order to compare the
morphological and biochemical features of control and "differentiated" cells. Most of the data presented here have
been obtained 3 days after treatment, because at this time
the differentiated phenotype for the most part becomes irreversibly fixed.

Table 4. Incidence of Tumors after Subcutaneous Injection of Control and "Differentiated" Neuroblastoma Cells

Treatment	No. of Animals	Incidence of Tumors (% of total)
Control cells treated or without solvent	30	100
RO20-1724	15	40
PGE$_1$	15	25
PGE$_1$ + RO20-1724	16	0

Cells (10^5) were plated in the Falcon plastic dishes (60 mm) and treated with drugs 24 hours later. 4-(-3-butoxy-4-methoxybenzyl)-2-imidazolidinone (RO20-1724, 200 μg/ml) and prostaglandin (PG)E$_1$ (10 μg/ml) were added individually or in combination. After 4 days of incubation the un-treated and treated-cells (0.25 x 10^6) were injected sub-cutaneously into male A/J mice (6 - 8 weeks of age). The cell viability in control and drug-treated culture was 90 - 95%. The data were presented from a previous publication (25).

Ultrastructural Changes

Some of the features of control cells which include the presence of dense chromatin materials at the periphery of nucleus, fewer mitochondria, golgi apparatus and rough endoplasmic reticulum (RER) in the cytoplasm resemble undifferentiated nerve cells, whereas others such as the presence of distinct nucleolus and catecholamine granules (CG) resemble mature neurons. Table 5 shows that in "differentiated" cells (3 days after treatment) the number of mitochondria and golgi apparatus increased, chromatin materials largely disappeared. These features resemble mature neurons. No change in RER and CG were seen. Sodium butyrate-treated cells also showed an increase in the number of mitochondria and golgi apparatus (3 days after treatment), but other features were similar to those of control cells. Thus except for rarity of RER, the "differentiated" cells for the most part resemble mature neurons.

Tyrosine Hydroxylase (TH)

Tyrosine hydroxylase, a rate limiting enzyme in the biosynthesis of catecholamine is present in neuroblastoma clones (8, 10). Some analogs of cyclic AMP and papaverine (PDE inhibitor), increased (Table 6) the TH activity by 30- to 50-fold (26, 27). Dibutyryl cyclic AMP also increased the TH activity in a neuroblastoma clone which did not show morphological differentiation. Morphologically differentiated neuroblastoma cells induced by x-ray (28), serum free medium (29) and cytosine arabinoside (30) did not show any change in TH level (27, 30). Butyric acid, which inhibits cell division without causing morphological differentiation (16) also increased the enzyme activity (27). Butyric acid increased (31) cyclic AMP level by about 2-fold (Table 7). These data suggest that morphological differentiation and TH activity are independently regulated, and cyclic AMP may be involved in the regulation of TH activity.

Choline Acetyltransferase (ChA) and Acetylcholinesterase (AChE)

The ChA which synthesizes acetylcholine was present in the neuroblastoma cells exclusively or in association with TH activity. Table 8 shows that dibutyryl cyclic AMP, PGE$_1$ or RO20-1724, papaverine, 8-benzylthio cyclic AMP, sodium butyrate, x-irradiation or 5' AMP markedly increased ChA activity. The time of increased enzyme activity coincided

218

Table 5. Ultrastructural Changes in Differentiated Neuroblastoma Cells Induced by Dibutyryl Cyclic AMP (DBcAMP)

		Control	DBcAMP	Na butyrate
Nuclear		1) Distinct nucle-olus	Distinct Nucleolus	Distinct nucleolus
Changes		2) Dense chromatin materials (Ch) at the periphery	Dense Ch largely disappear	Dense Ch at the periphery
Cytoplasmic		1) Rarity of rough endoplasmic reticulum (rER)	Rarity of rER	Rarity of rER
Changes		2) Fewer Mitochondria (MI) and golgi apparatus (GA)	Marked increase in MI and moderately increase in GA	Abundance of MI and GA
		3) Abundance of "finger-like" projections (FP) on cell surface	Fewer FP	Abundance of FP
		4) Variable No. of catecholamine granules (CG)	Variable No. CG, no change	Variable No. of CG, no change

Dibutyryl cyclic AMP (0.5 mM) and Sodium butyrate (0.5 mM)
were added to each culture 24 hours after plating. Fresh
growth medium and drug solutions were changed 2 days after
treatment and cells were removed by a rubber policeman for
electron microscopic study. Several grids of control and
treated cells were examined and the summary of nuclear and
cytoplasmic changes was presented.

Table 6. Tyrosine Hydroxylase Activity and Differentiation of Mouse Neuroblastoma Cells in Culture

Treatment	Tyrosine Hydroxylase pmol product/30 min/10^6 cells
Control, log phase	15.1 ± 1.9*
Control, confluent phase	11.2 ± 0.7
Serum free medium	17.3 ± 0.4
Dibutyryl cyclic AMP (0.25 mM)	473 ± 17
8-methylthio cyclic AMP (0.3 mM)	587 ± 9
Papaverine (0.13 mM)	977 ± 46
Sodium butyrate (0.5 mM)	300 ± 12
X-irradiation (600 rads)	14 ± 2
X-irradiation (600 rads) plus Sodium Butyrate (0.5 mM)	764 ± 90

*Standard deviation

NBP_2 clone was used in this study. This clone has both tyrosine hydroxylase (TH) and choline acetyltransferase.
Neuroblastoma (0.5 x 10^6) were treated with x-rays 24 hrs.
later. The data were taken from a previous publication
(26). Each value represents an average of at least 4
samples.

Table 7. Effect of Various Agents on the Cyclic AMP Level
of Mouse Neuroblastoma Cells in Culture

Treatment	Cyclic AMP Level pmol/mg protein
Control	12 ± 1.5*
5-bromodeoxyuridine (5.0 μM)	21.8 ± 1.7
Serum Free Medium	22.5 ± 2.2
X-irradiation (600 rads)	13.5 ± 1.8
6-thioguanine (0.5 μM)	14.4 ± 2.1
6-mercaptopurine (0.5 μM)	13.9 ± 2.1
2-aminopurine (5.0 μM)	10.3 ± 1.4
Butyric Acid (0.5 mM)	22.0 ± 3.2
Prostaglandin E_1 (10 μg/ml)	47.1 ± 5.3
4-(3-butoxy-4-methoxybenzyl)-2-imidazolidinone (200 μg/ml)	42.3 ± 4.4
Theophylline (0.5 mM)	11.0 ± 2.4

*Standard deviation

Cells (0.5×10^6) of neuroblastoma clone $NBA_2(1)$ were plated in large Falcon plastic flasks (75 cm^2) and various
treatments were given individually 24 hours later. Fresh
growth medium and drug solution were changed 2 days after
treatment and cyclic AMP level was analysed 3 days after
treatment. Each value represented an average of 6 - 10
samples.

Table 8. Effect of Various Agents on Choline Acetyltransferase Level of Neuroblastoma Cells

Treatment	Choline Acetyltransferase Activity (pmol/15 min/10^6 cells)
Control (Exponential)	260 ± 35*
Control (Confluent)	300 ± 34
Dibutyryl cyclic AMP (0.5 mM)	1300 ± 72
Prostaglandin E_1 (10 µg/ml)	880 ± 100
4-(3-butoxy-4-methoxybenzyl) -2-imidazolidinone (200 µg/ml)	1280 ± 160
Papaverine (25 µg/ml)	1220 ± 140
8-benzylthio, 3',5' cyclic AMP (400 µg/ml)	1080 ± 40
3',5' cyclic AMP (0.5mM)	301 ± 60
5' AMP (0.25 mM)	1320 ± 80
Butyric acid (0.5 mM)	760 ± 100
Gamma-aminobutyric Acid (0.5 mM)	240 ± 40
600 rads	1640 ± 144

*Standard deviation

Neuroblastoma cells (0.5×10^6) were plated in the Falcon plastic flasks (75 cm^2) and each drug was added 24 hours later. Each value represents an average of 6 - 8 samples.

with the time of inhibition of cell division (32). All of
the above agents inhibit cell division and all but sodium
butyrate, 3', 5' cyclic AMP and 5' AMP cause morphological
differentiation. These data indicate that the levels of
ChA and morphological differentiation are independently regulated and inhibition of cell division allows the expression of high level of ChA. Cyclic AMP may not be necessarily involved in the regulation of this enzyme. A similar
mechanism has been suggested for the regulation of AChE
(33).

Effect of Butyric Acid, Gamma-aminobutyric Acid and B-hydroxybutyric Acid

Butyric acid structurally resembles the neurobiologic-
ally active substances gamma-aminobutyric acid and B-hydroxybutyric acid. Butyric acid (sodium salt) inhibited
cell division without causing morphological differentiation. On removal of the drug three days after treatment,
cell division resumed (Figure 4). This is in contrast to
dibutyryl cyclic AMP-treated cells which do not resume cell
division after removal of the drug (17). Sodium butyrate
increased the levels of TH (27), ChA (32), AChE (33) and
COMT (34), whereas dibutyryl cyclic AMP increased the
levels of only the first three enzymes. Gamma-aminobutyric
acid and B-hydroxybutyric acid although structurally resemble butyric acid, had no effect on the growth of neuroblastoma cells. Therefore, our earlier suggestions (26)
that butyric acid may mimic the effect of a neurobio-
logically active substances like gamma-aminobutyric and B-
hydroxybutyric acid is not true, at least on the criteria
used in this study.

Levels of DNA, RNA and protein contents

Since a marked increase in the size of soma and nucleus
is seen during cyclic AMP-induced "differentiation" of
neuroblastoma cells, changes in the total contents of nucleic acid and protein were investigated 3 days after treatment. Table 9 shows the total DNA contents of "differentiated" cells markedly decreased (35), but total RNA and protein contents increased by about two to three fold. The
pronounced reduction in the DNA content per cell is interpreted as an evidence that most of cells accumulate in the
G_1-phase of the cycle. An increase in RNA and protein contents is consistent with the observation made during

223

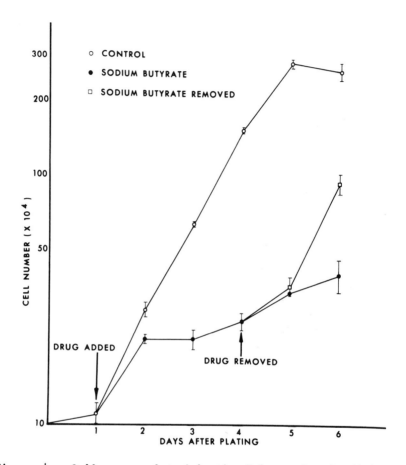

Figure 4. Cells were plated in the Falcon plastic dishes
(60 mm) and butyric acid (sodium salt) and gamma-aminobutyric acid (0.5 mM) were added separately 24 hours after
plating. The cell number was counted by a Coulter counter.
The growth pattern of gamma-aminobutyric acid-treated cells
was similar to that of controls and therefore, not shown in
the Figure. In one group of dishes sodium butyrate was
removed and fresh growth medium was added. In another
group of dishes, fresh growth medium and sodium butyrate
were replaced at the same time. The growth medium in control and gamma-aminobutyric acid was also changed. Each
point represents an average of 6 - 8 samples. The vertical
bars are standard deviations.

Table 9. Total DNA, RNA and protein contents in cyclic AMP-induced "differentiated" mouse neuroblastoma cells in culture

Treatment	DNA (pg/cell)	RNA (pg/cell)	Protein (pg/cell)
Control	13.3 ± 1.5*	15.3 ± 1.0	500 ± 29
DBcAMP	6.6 ± 0.6	33.6 ± 2.5	1580 ± 122
PGE$_1$	6.0 ± 1.6	24.4 ± 1.9	870 ± 47
RO20-1724	6.7 ± 1.2	33 ± 1.8	1016 ± 54
Na butyrate	5.3 ± 1.0	31.2 ± 3.9	1479 ± 111

*Standard deviation

Cells (0.5×10^6) were plated in large Falcon plastic Flask (75 cm^2) and dibutyryl cyclic AMP (DBcAMP, 0.5 mM), prostaglandin (PG)E$_1$ (10 μg/ml), 4-(-3-butoxy-4-methoxybenzyl)-2-imidazolidinone (RO20-1724, 200 μg/ml), and sodium butyrate (Na butyrate, 0.5 mM) were added separately 24 hrs. later. The total nucleic acid and protein contents were assayed 3 days after treatment. Each value represents an average of 4 to 6 samples. The data were presented from a previous publication (35).

Table 10. Total DNA, RNA and Protein Contents in
"Differentiated" mouse Neuroblastoma Cells (NBE⁻(R)) in
Culture Induced by non-cyclic AMP Agents

Treatment	DNA (pg/cell)	RNA (pg/cell)	Protein (pg/cell)
Control	19.8 ± 2.7*	26 ± 1.3	152 ± 13
SFM	23.8 ± 2.3	65 ± 9.0	180 ± 12
6-thioguanine	25.4 ± 3.5	79 ± 12.0	346 ± 7.0
5-BrdU	7 ± 1.5	50 ± 3.4	343 ± 34
X-ray	62 ± 13.8	153 ± 27.0	768 ± 39

*Standard deviations

Cells (0.5 - 1 x 10^6) were plated in large Falcon plastic
flasks and serum free medium (SFM), 5-bromodeoxyuridine
(5-BrdU, 5 µM), 6-thioguanine (0.5 µM) and x-ray (1200 rads)
were given separately 24 hr later. The total DNA, RNA and
protein contents were analysed 3 days after treatment.
Each value represents an average of 5 - 8 samples.

differentiation and maturation of mammalian neurons. Sodium butyrate treated cells were also accumulated in the G_1-phase; however, the expression of differentiated phenotype did not occur indicating that inhibition of cell division is not sufficient for the expression of morphological differentiation.

Level of PDE

The morphologically "differentiated" cells induced by dibutyryl cyclic AMP, PGE_1 and RO20-1724 have a four-fold higher cyclic AMP level than the control cells. The PDE activity in the "differentiated" cell increased by about three-fold and did not return to a control level when the drug was removed 3 days after treatment. Dibutyryl cyclic AMP and PGE_1 caused an increase in PDE activity 2 hours after treatment; however, RO20-1724 inhibited the PDE activity by about 50 percent of controls at this time (Figure 5). RO20-1724 later increased the PDE activity to the same level as that by dibutyryl cyclic AMP. Theophylline, butyric acid, 5' AMP, x-irradiation and confluency did not change the PDE level. Except for butyric acid, none of the above agents change the cyclic AMP level. Thus generally, a high level of cyclic AMP is associated with a high level of PDE. A working hypothesis is proposed (36) that an increase in the levels of cyclic AMP and PDE is associated with the differentiation of neuroblastoma cells; the reverse may be true during malignant transformation of nerve cells. Other workers have shown (37, 38) that in fibroblasts cyclic AMP acts as an inducer of PDE.

"Differentiated" Cells induced by Non-cyclic AMP Agents

Some non-cyclic AMP agents such as x-ray (28), serum free medium (29), cytosine arabinoside (30), 5-BrdU (39) and 6-thioguanine (40) cause morphological differentiation similar to that produced by cyclic AMP (17 - 19). Therefore, the question arose whether they produce morphological differentiation by increasing the intracellular level of cyclic AMP or they produce changes similar to those produced by cyclic AMP. Table 7 shows that serum free medium and 5-BrdU increased the cyclic AMP by about two-fold, whereas, x-ray and 6-thioguanine did not. In addition, sodium butyrate increased the cyclic AMP level without allowing the expression of differentiated phenotype. Table 10 shows that the total RNA and protein contents markedly

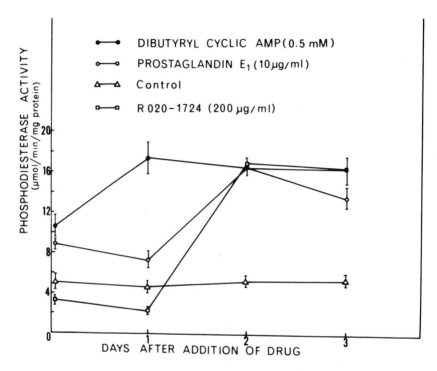

Figure 5. Neuroblastoma cells (0.5×10^6) were plated in large Falcon plastic flasks (75 cm^2). Dibutyryl cyclic AMP prostaglandin E$_1$ and 4-(3-butoxy-4-methoxybenzyl)-2-imidazolidione (RO20-1724) were added individually for a period of 2 hours, 1 day, 2 days, and 3 days. Fresh growth medium and drug solution were added 2 days after treatment with drug. The cyclic AMP phosphodiesterase (PDE) activity was analyzed according to the procedure described previously (16). Each value represents an average of 8 - 10 samples. The vertical bars are standard deviations (36).

increased in "differentiated" cells. The DNA content of
BrdU-treated cells decreased by about 66 percent of controls, indicating that most of the cells were accumulated
in the G_1-phase of the cycle, whereas in x-irradiated cells
it increased by about 3-fold indicating that most of cells
were arrested in the G_2-phase and/or polyploid cells expressed differentiated phenotype. X-irradiation causes po-
lyploidy in most mammalian cell cultures; thus the expression of differentiated phenotype and some of its associated
functions in polyploid cells is consistent with the fact
that some mammalian neurons are tetraploids (41-43). The
DNA contents of 6-thioguanine (TG) and serum free medium
(SFM) treated cells did not change indicating that the relative distribution of cells in various phases of the cell
cycle was unchanged.

Comparative Features of Morphologically "Differentiated" Cells Induced by Cyclic AMP and Non-cyclic AMP Agents

The morphologically "differentiated" induced by cyclic
AMP and non-cyclic AMP agents differ in some respects. In
cyclic AMP-induced "differentiated" cells a high PDE level
was associated with a high cyclic AMP level. DNA content
decreased, but the RNA and protein contents increased. The
morphologically "differentiated" cells induced by non-cyclic AMP agents, showed only some of the above changes and
they too were variable depending upon the agent used. SFM
and 5-BrdU increased the cyclic AMP level, but x-ray and 6-
TG did not. The DNA content increased in x-irradiated
cells, decreased in 5-BrdU-treated cells, and did not
change in SFM- and 6-TG-treated cells. The total RNA and
protein increased in cells treated with all non-cyclic AMP
agents. The TH activity did not change after x-irradiation
(34). The AChE increased after x-irradiation (33) and SFM
(30). The ChA increased after treatment with x-irradiation
(32), 6-TG (40), 5-BrdU (39) and SFM (29).

Since sodium butyrate increases the cyclic AMP level
without causing morphological differentiation, and x-irradiation and 6-TG cause morphological differentiation without increasing the cyclic AMP level it is concluded that
neither the elevation of cyclic AMP is always sufficient
for the expression of differentiated phenotype nor

the expression of differentiated phenotype always requires the elevation of cyclic AMP. Nevertheless, cyclic AMP may be a better tool to study the problem of differentiation of neuroblastoma cells than other agents because it is a naturally occuring substance and unlike non-cyclic AMP agents induces most of the differentiating functions. Data presented here substantiate the previous hypothesis that the morphological "differentiation" and neural enzymes appears to be independently regulated.

The neuroblastoma cells may have some limitation, when used as an experimental model of undifferentiated nerve cells because they possess some features of mature neurons. The "differentiated" cells induced by cyclic AMP may also have some limitations when used as an experimental model of mature neurons because they maintain some features of undifferentiated cells. In spite of some limitations neuroblastoma cell culture provides relatively a simple model to study the various aspects of neurobiology such as mechanism of differentiation, function of individual neurons, regulation of neural enzymes and mechanism of drug action.

Acknowledgement

This work was supported by USPH NS09230, IP02-CA-12247-01AL and DRG-1182 from Daymon Runyon Memorial Fund for Cancer Research. I thank Drs. J. E. Pike of UpJohn Company, H. Sheppard of Hoffamann-La-Roach and R. K. Robins of ICN Nucleic Acid Research Institute for generous supply of prostaglandins, RO20-1724 and 8-substituted analogs of cyclic AMP.

References

1. R. R. Burk, Nature 219, 1272 (1968).
2. W. L. Ryan and Heidrick, Science 16, 1484 (1968).
3. A. W. Hsie and T. T. Puck, Proc. Natl. Acad. Sci., U.S. 68, 358 (1971).
4. G. S. Johnson, R. M. Friedman and I. Pastan, Proc. Natl. Acad. Sci., U.S. 68, 425 (1971).
5. J. R. Sheppard, Proc. Natl. Acad. Sci., U.S. 68,1316 (1971).
6. K. N. Prasad, Cancer Res. 31, 1457 (1971).
7. A. Sakamoto and K. N. Prasad, Cancer Res. 32, 532 (1972)
8. G. Augusti-Tocco and G. Sato, Proc. Natl. Acad. Sci.,

U.S. <u>64</u>, 311 (1969).

9. A. Blume, F. Gilbert, S. Wilson, J. Farber, R. Rosenberg and M. Nirenberg, <u>Proc. Natl. Acad. Sci.</u>, U.S. <u>67</u>, 786 (1970).

10. K. N. Prasad, B. Mandal, J. C. Waymire, G. J. Lees, A. Vernadakis and N. Weiner, <u>Nature</u> (in press).

11. A. Amano, E. Richelson and M. Nirenberg, <u>Proc. Natl. Acad. Sci.</u>, U.S. <u>69</u>, 258 (1972).

12. K. N. Prasad, B. Mandal and S. Kumar, <u>J. Pediat.</u> (in press).

13. T. Posternak, E. W. Sutherland and W. F. Hemion, <u>Biochem. Biophys. Acta.</u> <u>65</u>, 558 (1962).

14. R. W. Butcher, <u>Adv. Biochem. Psychopharmacol</u> <u>3</u>, 173 (1970).

15. H. Sheppard and G. Wiggan, <u>Molecular Pharmacol</u>, <u>7</u>, 111 (1971).

16. N. D. Goldberg, D. W. Lust, R. F. O'Dea, S. Wei and A. G. O'Toole, <u>Adv. Biochem. Pharmacol.</u> <u>3</u>, 67 (1970).

17. K. N. Prasad and A. W. Hsie, <u>Nature New Biol.</u> <u>233</u>, 141 (1971).

18. K. N. Prasad, <u>Nature New Biol.</u> <u>236</u>, 49 (1972).

19. K. N. Prasad and J. R. Sheppard, <u>Expt. Cell Res.</u> <u>73</u>, 436 (1972).

20. K. N. Prasad, <u>Proc. Soc. Exp. Biol. Med.</u> <u>140</u>, 126 (1972).

21. P. Furmanski, D. J. Silverman and M. Lubin, <u>Nature</u> <u>233</u>, 413 (1971).

22. A. G. Gilman and M. Nirenberg, <u>Nature</u> <u>234</u>, 356 (1971).

23. J. G. Hardman, J. W. Davis and E. W. Sutherland, <u>J. Biol. Chem.</u> <u>244</u>, 6354 (1969).

24. K. N. Prasad, <u>Cytobiologie</u> <u>5</u>, 272 (1972).

25. K. N. Prasad, <u>Cytobiologie</u> (in press).

26. J. C. Waymire, N. Weiner and K. N. Prasad, <u>Proc. Natl. Acad. Sci.</u>, U.S. <u>69</u>, 2241 (1972).

27. K. N. Prasad, J. C. Waymire and N. Weiner, <u>Exptl. Cell Res.</u> <u>74</u>, 110 (1972).

28. K. N. Prasad, <u>Nature</u> <u>234</u>, 471 (1971).

29. N. W. Seeds, A. G. Gilman, T. Amano and M. W. Nirenberg, <u>Proc. Natl. Acad. Sci.</u>, U.S. <u>66</u>, 160 (1970).

30. J. R. Kates, R. Winterton and K. Schlessinger, <u>Nature</u> <u>229</u>, 345 (1971).

31. K. N. Prasad and S. Kumar, (in preparation).

32. K. N Prasad and B. Mandal, (in preparation).

33. K. N. Prasad and A. Vernadakis, <u>Exptl. Cell Res.</u> <u>70</u>,

27 (1972).

34. K. N. Prasad and B. Mandal, Exptl. Cell Res. 74, 532 (1972).

35. K. N. Prasad, S. Kumar, K. Gilmar and A. Vernadakis, Biochem. Biophys. Res. Commun. (in press).

36. K. N. Prasad and S. Kumar, Proc. Soc. Exp. Biol. Med. (in press).

37. M. D'Armiento, G. S. Johnson and I. Pastan, Proc. Natl. Acad. Sci., U.S. 69, 459 (1972).

38. V. Maganiello and M. Vaughan, Proc. Natl. Acad. Sci., U.S. 69, 269-273 (1972).

39. D. Shubert and F. Jacobs, Proc. Natl. Acad. Sci., U.S. 67, 247 (1970).

40. K. N. Prasad, B. Mandal and S. Kumar, (in preparation)

41. H. A. Muller, Naturwiss 49, 243 (1962).

42. A. A. Kusch and V. N. Yarygin, Tistologia 7, 228 (1965).

43. L. W. Lapham, Science, 159, 310 (1968).

DISCUSSION

B. Weiss, Philadelphia: Have you noticed any increase in synaptic connections between the cells in response to dibutyryl cyclic AMP?

K.N. Prasad, University of Colorado, Denver: I have not done electron microscopy in detail, therefore I can't answer your question at this time.

R. Sharma, VA Hospital, Memphis: Dr. Prasad, this question is not only directed at you but perhaps anybody else who might care to comment on it. Has anybody tested butyryic anhydride? And can butyryic anhydride imitate the action of butyric acid?

K.N. Prasad: I haven't done it.

G. Krishna, National Institutes of Health: Have you studied whether catecholamine uptake is increased after differentiation?

K.N. Prasad: At this time we are doing this experiment and at least in the control culture, it seems that the uptake of catecholamine is insensitive to cocaine, which is supposed to block the uptake in normal mature neurons.

A. Berg, Medical College of Pennsylvania: We have obtained data from *in vivo* studies which substantiate Dr. Prasad's experimental systems as models of normal neuronal differentiation. We have measured the distribution of cyclic AMP across the cerebral cortex of rats of different ages. As others have reported, we find that cyclic AMP levels in this cortex increase from birth to

233

a peak by 30 to 60 days of age. We have now completed measurements on older animals and find that cortical cyclic AMP levels fall to values only 20% of the maximum by age 6 months and thereafter maintain this adult level over the next year. Thus if cyclic AMP is involved normally in neural differentiation, its continued presence at very high concentrations appears to be unnecessary for maintenance of the differentiated state.

J. Neumann, Boston University: I believe you said that the appearance of some of the enzymatic markers of differentiation preceded the inhibition of growth or cell division after dibutyryl cAMP treatment.

K.N. Prasad: Right.

J. Neumann: Does this include the activity of, for instance, cholinesterase and if sok has this enzyme's activity peaked by the time cell division has stopped?

K.N. Prasad: That's correct. It seems that a significant increase in neural enzymes are seen one day after treatment, but a maximal elevation coincides with the time of inhibition of cell division.

G. Krishna: I want to ask you. Have you ever used tributyryl AMP for a control for cyclic dibutyryl AMP or cyclic AMP?

K.N. Prasad: No, I haven't.

G. Krishna: It's really a better control because butyric acid release may be extremely small in comparison to dibutyryl cyclic AMP.

K.N. Prasad: I agree with you. However, we routinely used inhibitors of phosphodiesterase and, therefore it may not be necessary.

P.A. Galand, Free University, Brussels, Belgium:
Did I understand you, when you showed the data on DNA
content? Was a 2-fold decrease in mean DNA content,
in "differentiated" cells?

K.N. Prasad: Yes.

P.A. Galand: At what time was this?

K.N. Prasad: Three days after treatment, when
cell divison has stopped.

P.A. Galand: And did you observe any wave of
mitotic activity in the days before this time?

K.N. Prasad: No. The growth inhibition produced
by cyclic AMP is for the most part irreversible.

P.A. Galand: Because if you conclude that this indicates
that they are in G_1 mainly, this would also indicate that
"nondifferentiated" cells are in G_2.

K.N. Prasad: No, I am simply saying that the cyclic
AMP induced, "differentiated" cells had DNA content
of about 50% of control, which indicates that most of these
cells were in the G_1 stage of the cell cycle; however,
by blocking the cells in G_1 does not necessarily mean
that the morphological differentiation will be expressed,
since butyric acid treated cells also accumulated in
the G_1 phase, but did not express morphological
differentiation.

P.A. Galand: Since Dr. Prasad said that the 50%
reduction in DNA content in the cyclic AMP-induced,
differentiated cells indicates that those cells are in G_1,
does he imply therefore, that most of the "undifferentiated"
neuroblastoma cells (before treatment with cAMP) are
in the G_2 phase of the cell cycle?

K.N. Prasad: We do not know what fraction of control cells are in the G_2 phase. I see your concern, because the DNA content is about half of the control. In case of diploid cells, one would expect that the DNA content of these cells should have been slightly higher than reported here. However, neuroblastoma cells are aneuploids; therefore we may not get the value which might be expected if cells were diploid.

T.T. Puck, University of Colorado: Did you measure the plating efficiency of your cultures after treatment with these various agents?

K.N. Prasad: The plating efficiency of all our clones is very poor and therefore such experiments, although very important cannot be performed at this time.

T.T. Puck: Under these circumstances, I think then, some of your conclusions have to be regarded as extremely tentative. For example, the apparent loss of the ability to produce a tumor might be due to a decrease in the number of reproducing cells. The ability to transport certain vital dyes does not imply the ability of the cells to reproduce. If these cells always lose reproductive potential, as a result of such treatment, the fact would be an extremely interesting phenomenon. It might mean that differentiation in this neuroblastoma cell must be accompanied by loss of the power to reproduce, as indeed happens in the normal tissue.

K.N. Prasad: I share your caution at this time. However, those cells which have been treated with cyclic AMP for the most part do not resume cell division. This is consistent with the nerve differentiation. If neuroblastoma cells are indeed "differentiated", we expect the loss of reproductive capacity. The data which we have obtained thus far indicate that the "differentiated" cells for the most part are irreversible, provided the drug is allowed to remain in the medium for at least 3 days. If their response to cyclic AMP changes at a later date, I cannot predict.

E.E. Smith, Boston University School of Medicine: I have a comment and then a question. First of all, some of our results of treating KB cells with cyclic AMP parallel the results of treatment of neuroblastoma with dibutyryl cyclic AMP, namely, we saw no decrease in agglutinability. If anything, there was an increase. Secondly, we saw a distinct change in the nucleus. One question I'd like to ask is how long you followed these cells to measure irreversibility.

K.N. Prasad: 4-6 days after removal of drug.

E.E. Smith: How long did you let the cells grow after you had removed the drug?

K.N. Prasad: This question has been asked again and again, and I will do more systematic study when I go back. We have observed differentiated culture up to 10 days after various treatments. We see that as a function of time the "differentiated" cells probably start to die, as evidenced by a few floating cells. But the rate of death is extremely slow. The differentiated morphology is maintained in culture for a relatively long time. The death of "differentiated" cells is consistent with the fact that the mature neurons can't be maintained in the culture for a longer period.

S. Strada, University of Texas: Is calcium essential for the formation of neurites, and have you measured protein kinase activity in these cells?

K.N. Prasad: Well, we did the calcium study, but I don't know whether it is conclusive. We added cyclic AMP agents in the calcium free medium containing dialyzed serum. The expression of differentiated phenotype occurred in a manner similar to that observed in the normal growth medium containing cyclic AMP agents.

CYCLIC AMP AND THE EXPRESSION OF DIFFERENTIATED PROPERTIES IN VITRO

Philip Furmanski and Martin Lubin
Department of Microbiology
Dartmouth Medical School

Abstract: Dibutyryl cyclic AMP acts on mouse neuroblastoma cells in a number of ways: it inhibits the DNA synthesis produced by addition of serum to serum-starved cells; when added to growing cells, it depresses incorporation of thymidine and deoxycytidine into DNA; it also depresses transport of thymidine and deoxycytidine, but not sufficiently to account for the observed degree of inhibition of incorporation; treated cells are as tumorigenic as untreated cells; and induction of neurites is rapid and unrelated to depression of DNA synthesis.

INTRODUCTION

Several years ago, Ballard and Tomkins (1) reported that dexamethasone increased the adhesiveness of fibroblasts to culture dishes. Their work prompted us to see if any of a variety of hormones might induce morphological changes in mouse neuroblastoma cells. We found that dibutyryl cyclic AMP, which had been shown to alter the morphology of fibroblastic tumor cells (2,3), induced the formation of long processes, called "neurites" (4). Dibutyryl cyclic AMP also increased the level of acetylcholinesterase activity. Similar findings were simultaneously

239

reported by Prasad and Hsie (5).

The C1300 tumor was introduced into in vitro culture by Augusti-Tocco and Sato (6), and Klebe and Ruddle (7). It originated in the Jackson Laboratories, and was classified for years as a "round cell" tumor. These investigators described many of its neural properties, and subsequently others reported that removal of serum (8), or addition of 5-BrdU (9), resulted in neurite extension. The effect of serum removal on what has been called "morphological" and "biochemical" differentiation (induction of specific enzymes, such as acetylcholinesterase) is probably due to an increase in intracellular cyclic AMP levels (10).

The functional significance of neurites is not known. No synaptic connections have yet been found between adjacent C1300 cells, nor has an indisputable neuromuscular junction been demonstrated between a C1300 cell and a striated muscle cell, although evidence for some interaction between the two cell types has been found (11).

Outgrowth of neurites has been induced by dibutyryl cyclic AMP in freshly excised ganglia (12,13). This suggests that the induction of neurites by dibutyryl cyclic AMP in C1300 cells has a counterpart in the physiology of normal cells, and that the neurites of the mouse neuroblastoma may indeed prove to be capable of forming synaptic junctions if only the right conditions can be found.

RESULTS AND DISCUSSION

(1) Serum and dibutyryl cyclic AMP antagonism.

Since the omission of serum from the culture medium and the addition of dibutyryl cyclic AMP to complete medium produce similar changes in C1300 cells, we measured the effects of a range of concentrations of dibutyryl cyclic AMP and serum. We used both baby hamster kidney (BHK) and C1300 (clone NB60) cells.

BHK cells were grown in Dulbecco's Modified Eagle Medium supplemented with 15% calf serum, and then transferred to medium containing only 0.5% serum. After 72 hours, by which time cell division had ceased, incorporation of ^{3}H-thymidine was markedly depressed. More serum was added, and 22 to 26 hours later the cells went through a synchronous wave of incorporation of thymidine and subsequently divided. Cell numbers increased at a rate determined by the amount of serum added (Fig. 1). At a concentration of 0.25 mM, dibutyryl cyclic AMP enhanced the stimulatory effect of added serum, but at 2 mM, it inhibited.

Thymidine incorporation was also dependent on the concentrations of both serum and dibutyryl cyclic AMP. As with measurements of changes in cell number, low concentrations of dibutyryl cyclic AMP enhanced, and high concentrations inhibited the stimulatory effects of serum (Fig.2).

Similarly, when NB60 cells were incubated for 72 hours in medium containing 0.5% serum, addition of serum stimulated both DNA synthesis (Fig. 3) and cell division (data not shown). On the whole, our results are similar to those recently reported by others (14, 15, 16, 17). We find, however, that the relation between the effects of dibutyryl cyclic AMP and of serum is complex: stimulation or inhibition by dibutyryl cyclic AMP depends both on concentration and on cell type.

Although dibutyryl cyclic AMP in NB60 cells markedly inhibited incorporation of thymidine, it inhibited incorporation of leucine, glucosamine, and uridine only modestly (Table 1).

TABLE 1

Effect of Dibutyryl Cyclic AMP
On Macromolecular Synthesis in NB60 Cells

	Dibutyryl Cyclic AMP Concentration		
	0	0.2 mM	2 mM
^{3}H-thymidine	100*	49	1.9
^{3}H-uridine	100	89	20
^{3}H-leucine	100	95	85
^{3}H-glucosamine	100	98	82

Cells were incubated in medium containing
0.5% serum for three days. 10% serum and
dibutyryl cyclic AMP were added. After 24
hours radioactive substrates were added,
and two hours later cell samples were
processed for measurement of incorporation.

*All values are expressed as percent of con-
trols without dibutyryl cyclic AMP.

Rozengurt and Pardee (14) found that transport
of amino-isobutyrate and glutamine in CHO cells
was depressed by dibutyryl cyclic AMP, and
Hauschka et al. (18) reported a very marked inhibition of thymidine transport by dibutyryl
cyclic AMP in these same cells. To determine the
possible role of inhibition of transport in the
observed depression of incorporation of DNA precursors, we measured uptake of radioactive substrates in the TCA soluble and insoluble fractions of NB60 cells.

Dibutyryl cyclic AMP depressed transport of
both thymidine and deoxycytidine (Fig. 4). For
each substrate, incorporation was more strongly

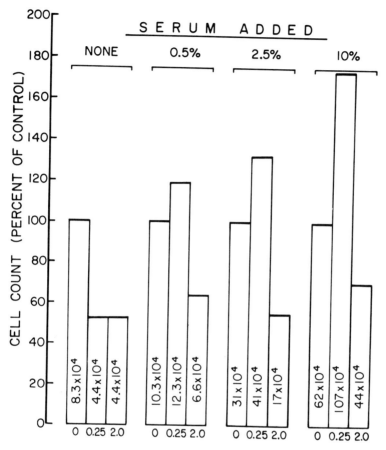

Fig. 1. BHK cells were incubated in medium with 0.5% serum for three days. Various amounts of serum and/or dibutyryl cyclic AMP were added, the cells were further incubated for three days, removed from the dishes by trypsinization, and counted in quadruplicate. Numbers within rectangles refer to cell counts per 30 cm^2 dish. At each serum concentration, the value for cell number shown on the ordinate is normalized to that for the culture without dibutyryl cyclic AMP, taken as 100%.

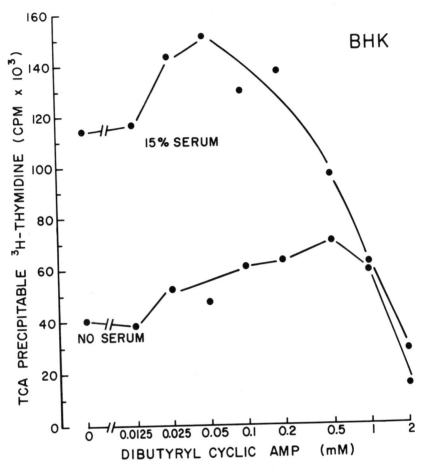

Fig. 2. BHK cells were incubated in medium containing 0.5% serum for three days. Serum and/or dibutyryl cyclic AMP were then added. 24 hours later ^{3}H-thymidine (2 μC/ml; 6.7 C/mmole) was added. Two hours later cell samples were processed to measure incorporation into trichloroacetic acid (TCA) precipitable material. They were washed three times with cold 10% TCA, once with phosphate buffered saline, and then taken up in Lowry Reagent C for counting.

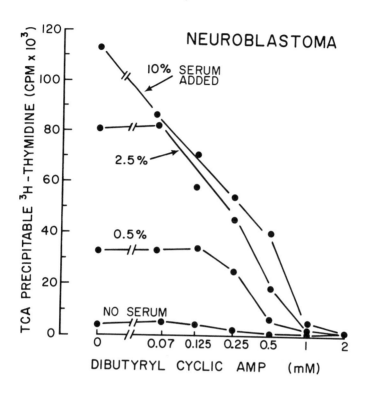

Fig. 3. NB60 cells were incubated for three days in medium containing 0.5% serum. Experimental details are the same as those in Fig. 2.

inhibited than was transport, although in the case of ^{3}H-thymidine, the difference was not pronounced until eight hours or more after the addition of dibutyryl cyclic AMP. Inhibition of transport, therefore, is not large enough to account completely for the observed inhibition of incorporation. In an experiment with ^{3}H-deoxyguanosine, we similarly found greater inhibition of incorporation than of transport.

The mechanism by which dibutyryl cyclic AMP depresses thymidine incorporation is not known. Cells deprived of serum are known to become arrested in G1 (19, 20). The results above (Fig. 1, 2, 3) indicate that dibutyryl cyclic AMP prevents serum-starved cells from synthesizing DNA (i.e., progressing from G1 to S) in response to addition of serum.

To determine if dibutyryl cyclic AMP would produce G1 arrest, we added it to growing cultures of NB60 cells; after 24 hours, new medium without dibutyryl cyclic AMP was added to release the cells from inhibition. DNA synthesis increased rapidly over the next three to six hours until, by 12 hours, the rate of synthesis was nearly equal to that of control cells. A significant increase in cell numbers was delayed, however, until about 36 hours after removal of dibutyryl cyclic AMP. These results and the findings of autoradiography described below suggest that most, but not all, of the cells were blocked or slowed in G1.

Induction of synthesis of some specific proteins of differentiated cells has been found to occur during the G1 phase of the cell cycle (21, 22). In addition, Blume et al.(23) reported that as neuroblastoma cells approached stationary phase (and probably became arrested in G1), acetylcholinesterase levels rose sharply. We suggest that induction of acetylcholinesterase and other enzymes after the addition of dibutyryl cyclic

246

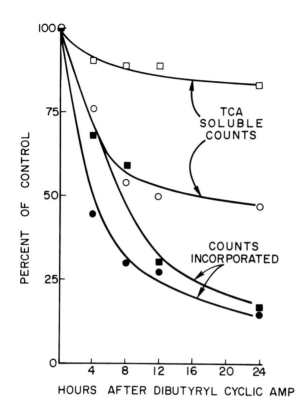

Fig. 4. Dibutyryl cyclic AMP was added to actively growing cultures of NB60 cells. At intervals ^{3}H-thymidine or ^{3}H-deoxycytidine (0.2 μC/ml; 0.1 C/mmole) was added. 60 minutes after each addition cells were rinsed three times with phosphate buffered saline at room temperature, and cold 5% TCA was added. Five minutes later, the TCA was removed and counted (TCA soluble fraction). After two more washes with cold TCA, cells were taken up in 0.5 M NaOH and counted (TCA insoluble fraction). Results of three experiments were averaged. Values are expressed as percent of measurements at zero time and are not corrected for increases in cell number, which, after 24 hours, amounted to about 30%. O , ■ , ^{3}H-thymidine; □ , ● , ^{3}H-deoxycytidine.

AMP to cultures of neuroblastoma cells need not necessarily be a specific effect of dibutyryl cyclic AMP, but may be only a secondary consequence of arrest in G1.

2. Tumorigenicity of NB60 cells treated with dibutyryl cyclic AMP.

The extent of differentiation of human neuroblastomas and the degree of malignancy of these tumors appear to be inversely correlated (24). We therefore examined the growth potential, in vivo, of NB60 cells which had first been induced in vitro to express their differentiated functions. Cells were incubated either in the absence of serum or in medium containing serum but with added dibutyryl cyclic AMP (1 mM). (After five days in the latter medium, cloning efficiency was reduced from 62% to 14%.) In both cases, cells showed no significant change in tumorigenicity compared to those taken from cultures (Table 2).

Treatment of tumor cells in culture with dibutyryl cyclic AMP has been reported (25, 26) to render them less reactive with concanavalin A and wheat germ agglutinin, plant lectins which possess the capacity to agglutinate tumor cells but not normal cells. We carried out experiments with NB60 and SV40-transformed Balb/3T3 cells and found that dibutyryl cyclic AMP had no significant effect on agglutination or hemadsorption (28) produced by concanavalin A. Neither did we observe any effect of serum deprivation of NB60 cells on agglutination or hemadsorption (Furmanski, Phillips, and Lubin, unpublished observations).

(3) DNA synthesis and induction of neurites.

The results in Fig. 4 show that dibutyryl cyclic AMP caused progressive inhibition of thymidine incorporation, with a half-maximal effect in six to eight hours. After 24 hours, incorporation was about 20% of the initial rate.

TABLE 2

Tumorigenicity of NB60 Cells
After Incubation With Dibutyryl Cyclic AMP

	Controls	With Dibutyryl Cyclic AMP
Number of mice with tumors/ Number inoculated	22/22	23/23
Average number of days from injection to appearance of tumor	16	14
Average number of days from injection to death	33	33

NB60 cells were incubated in medium with 15% calf serum and 1 mM dibutyryl cyclic AMP for five days. They were then removed from dishes and injected subcutaneously into strain A/J mice at 4×10^4 cells, an inoculum which is twice the minimal number of NB60 cells needed to produce progressively growing tumors consistently in 100% of the animals.

We have reported (4) that neurite extension reaches its maximum within 24 hours after addition of dibutyryl cyclic AMP. We recently found that if NB60 cells were sparsely seeded (less than 3,000 per cm^2), dibutyryl cyclic AMP induced pronounced neurite extension in as little as 60 to 90 minutes. When ^3H-thymidine is present in the medium for this same period, and the cells are fixed and prepared for autoradiography, a determination can be made of the fraction which shows both extended neurites and active DNA synthesis.

NB60 cells were seeded and allowed to grow for two days. Dibutyryl cyclic AMP and ^{3}H-thymidine (1 μC/ml; 6.7 C/mmole) were added. After 90 minutes, cells were washed once with phosphate buffered saline at room temperature, and were fixed for one hour in cold glutaraldehyde (1%, in half-strength phosphate buffered saline). Stripping film (Kodak AR10) was then applied and left in the dark for four weeks before photographic development. The results of this experiment show that at least 50% of the cells displayed both dark grains, due to the incorporation of ^{3}H-thymidine into DNA, and marked neurite extension (Fig. 5).

When cells were exposed to dibutyryl cyclic AMP for 24 hours, and then pulse-labeled for 90 minutes with ^{3}H-thymidine, the percent synthesizing DNA, as determined by autoradiography, dropped from the control value of close to 75% to about 25%. Those few cells which did show synthesis of DNA, moreover, had very much less grain density than the controls, probably due either to inhibition of transport of ^{3}H-thymidine or to a prolonged S phase.

To account for the arrest of most cells in G1 after prolonged exposure to dibutyryl cyclic AMP, we assume that cells initially in S and with extended neurites (Fig. 5, bottom) can progress through the cell cycle and accummulate in G1. Direct confirmation, however, needs to be obtained.

We conclude that morphological expression of differentiation (neurite extension) occurs very soon after the addition of dibutyryl cyclic AMP, and does not require inhibition of DNA synthesis.

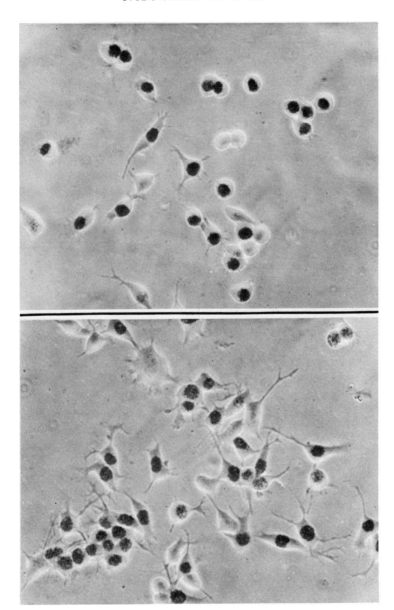

Fig. 5. Cells which had been synthesizing DNA
show dark nuclei. Top: control culture, without dibutyryl cyclic AMP. Bottom: 1 mM dibutyryl
cyclic AMP added.

REFERENCES

(1) P.L. Ballard and G.M. Tomkins, Nature 224 (1969) 344.

(2) G.S. Johnson, R. M. Friedman, and I. Pastan, Proc. US Nat. Acad. Sci. 68 (1971) 425.

(3) A.W. Hsie and T.T. Puck, Proc. US Nat. Acad. Sci. 68 (1971) 358.

(4) P. Furmanski, D.J. Silverman, and M. Lubin, Nature 233 (1971) 413.

(5) K.N. Prasad and A.W. Hsie, Nature New Biology 233 (1971) 141.

(6) G. Augusti-Tocco and G. Sato, Proc. US Nat. Acad. Sci. 64 (1969) 311.

(7) R.J. Klebe and F.H. Ruddle, J. Cell Biol. 43 (1969) 69a.

(8) N.W. Seeds, A.G. Gilman, T. Amano and M.W. Nirenberg, Proc. US Nat. Acad. Sci. 66 (1970) 160.

(9) D. Schubert and F. Jacob, Proc. US Nat. Acad. Sci. 67 (1970) 247.

(10) W. Frank, H.-J. Ristow and S. Zabel, European J. Biochem. 14 (1970) 392.

(11) A.J. Harris, S. Heinemann, D. Schubert and H. Tarakis, Nature 231 (1971) 296.

(12) D.B. Hier, B.G.W. Arnason and M. Young, Proc. US Nat. Acad. Sci. 69 (1972) 2268.

(13) F.J. Roisen, R.A. Murphy and W.G. Braden, Science 177 (1972) 809.

(14) E. Rozengurt and A.B. Pardee, J. Cell. Physiol. 80 (1972) 273.

(15) W. Frank, Exptl. Cell Res. 71 (1972) 238.

(16) J.E. Zimmerman and K. Raska, Nature New Biology 239 (1972) 145.

(17) J.E. Froehlich and M. Rachmeler, J. Cell Biol. 55 (1972) 19.

(18) P.V. Hauschka, L.P. Everhart and R.W. Rubin, Proc. US Nat. Acad. Sci. 69 (1972) 2542.

(19) R.R. Bürk, Exptl. Cell Res. 63 (1970) 309.

(20) G.D. Clark, M.G.P. Stoker, A. Ludlow and M. Thornton, Nature 227 (1970) 798.

(21) M. Cikes and S. Friberg, Jr., Proc. US Nat. Acad. Sci. 68 (1971) 566.

(22) D. Martin, Jr., G.M. Tomkins and D. Granner, Proc. US Nat. Acad. Sci. 62 (1969) 248.

(23) A. Blume, F. Gilbert, S. Wilson, J. Farber, R. Rosenberg and M. Nirenberg, Proc. US Nat. Acad. Sci. 67 (1970) 786.

(24) H. Cushing and S.B. Wolbach, Amer. J. Pathol. 3 (1927) 203.

(25) J.R. Sheppard, Proc. US Nat. Acad. Sci. 68 (1971) 1316.

(26) A.W. Hsie, C. Jones and T.T. Puck, Proc. US Nat. Acad. Sci. 68 (1971) 1648.

(27) P. Furmanski, P.G. Phillips and M. Lubin, Proc. Soc. Exp. Biol. and Med. 140 (1972) 216.

We acknowledge support by grants from the National Institute of Allergy and Infectious Diseases, U.S. Public Health Service (5-RO1 AI09288), the American Cancer Society (#E 577), and The Milheim Foundation (Project No. 72-17). P. Furmanski was the recipient of post-doctoral fellowships from the Damon Runyon Memorial Fund for Cancer Research (DRF-588) and the National Institutes of Health (2 FO2 CA41163). Janice Ratner rendered valuable assistance.

DISCUSSION

C. Zeilig, Vanderbilt University: Under exactly what conditions did you see the opposite effects of dibutyryl cyclic AMP, that is, the stimulation to which you alluded?

M. Lubin, Dartmouth Medical School: Are you referring to stimulation of thymidine incorporation?

C. Zeilig: Yes.

M. Lubin: These are conditions in which BHK cells are starved for three days in 0.5% serum, at which time the level of incorporation of thymidine was very low (Fig. 2). A low level of cyclic AMP was then added; 1) either when no serum was added back, and 2) serum with the cyclic AMP. Even though there was a very low level of incorporation, of thymidine, over the range from 0.025 mM all the way up to 1 mM dibutyryl cyclic AMP. Furmanski saw what looks to me like about a 50% stimulation. Then, at about 2 mM, there was a pronounced decline. On the other hand if he used 15% serum to stimulate the cells in the range again of 0.025 mM dibutyryl cyclic AMP with a peak stimulation occurring at about a 0.1 mM and then a decline thereafter, he saw stimulation of incorporation, so that by the time he reached 0.5 mM dibutyryl cyclic AMP there was now pronounced inhibition. There is the precaution to be taken in interpreting this, that in this experiment he did not measure effect on the transport of thymidine. Dr. Raska, in some very nice work which is now published in Nature, showed that in similar experiments, not only dibutyryl cyclic AMP, but AMP has effects on thymidine incorporation.

C. Zeilig: My second comment is just to describe some
of our experiences with DNA synthesis in synchronized
HeLa cells. We've been using phosphodiesterase inhibitors
to elevate cyclic AMP and measuring the effects of this
compound on cyclic AMP levels and the length of S phase.
We find very little effect of this compound on the length
of S phase. However, when we do autoradiograms, we
do see a decreased grain count. When we measure total
DNA synthesis, find again very little effect on the rate of
total DNA synthesis, and the major effect that we have seen
is a pronounced lengthening of the G_2 phase of the cell
cycle.

J.H. Robinson, Imperial Cancer Research Fund London:
I was very struck by the effect of serum deprivation on
your cells. Is this a specific serum deprivation effect
or do you think it's a general nutrient deprivation effect?
That is, have you tested the effect of removing any of the
nutrients from the medium on differentiation of your cells?

M. Lubin: No, we haven't. What did you have in mind?

J.H. Robinson: An amino acid, for example.

M. Lubin: No, you mean such as a isoleucine which
might arrest cell in G_1?

J.H. Robinson: No.

I. Pastan, National Institutes of Health: The starvation
experiments were done in a medium supplemented with
amino acid so that the major effect would be the deprivation
of proteins and perhaps other things present in serum.

M. Lubin: Yes, this is a complete medium except for
serum.

J.H. Robinson: I wasn't suggesting that the medium
wasn't complete. I was just wondering whether you tested

the effects of withdrawing other things with serum present.

M. Lubin: No, we have not. And that would be interesting to do.

K.N. Prasad, University of Colorado: First, I would like to caution you, for no conclusion can be made regarding tumorgenicity by using one clone and only dibutyryl cyclic AMP. I'd like to ask whether you measure the morphological "differentiation" at the time you injected the cells into the animal, and if so to what extent was the "differentiation", that is, how many cells have neurites?

M. Lubin: They were extensive. I don't immediately have the data on what percent of cells in the population had neurites, but judging from other experiments I would guess well over 60% or 70%. This was after 5 days of treatment and they were removed in Dr. Furmanski's experiments, with EDTA in calcium, magnesium free, phosphate buffered saline. I don't think in those experiments he measured enzyme induction. I should like to ask Dr. Prasad how his cells were removed. Were they removed with EDTA, or were they removed with trypsin?

K.N. Prasad: They were removed with 0.25 viokase.

M. Lubin: Perhaps therein lies the difference.

K.N. Prasad: Another point which appears to be of some controversy and is important as well, is the relationship of inhibition of cell division and neurite formation. I think by using an asynchronous cell population as we are using, it can't be solved. To get a better answer, it is essential that we establish the above relationship in a synchronous cell population and on an individual cell basis. Grossly, it appears that the induction of morphological "differentiation", as defined by neurite formation, occurs prior to inhibition of cell division. This is also supported by the fact that Schubert and Jacob have reported 5 BudR causes differentiation at a concentration which doesn't inhibit DNA synthesis. The reason this concerns me is that fibroblasts treated with dibutyryl cyclic AMP are more adherent, therefore more difficult to remove with trypsin, and if indeed the length of trypsin treatment does affect the viability of the cells or some function of the cells, this may be a variable that people should think a bit about.

M. Lubin: May I interject a word, because, although I know that Dr. Furmanski removed cells with EDTA and then injected them into mice, I cannot remember if he carried out similar experiments with cells removed by trypsin. (Authors' note: These experiments were carried out and no change in tumorigenicity was found.)

I. Pastan: The reason this concerns me is that fibroblasts treated with dibutyryl cylic AMP are more adherent, therefore more difficult to remove with trypsin. If indeed the length of trypsin treatment does affect the viability of the cells or some function of the cells, this may be a variable that people should think a bit about.

G.N. Gill, University of California: Do you have additional information in terms of oncogenicity of the cells treated with cyclic AMP when injected into animals treated with cyclic AMP or with something which raises it at the same time. That is, can you inhibit the killing action by reproducing in the animal the same situation as in tissue culture?

M. Lubin: I don't. I believe that's been tried with negative results, but perhaps Dr. Pastan knows of some work where treatment of animals with cyclic AMP affected tumor growth.

I. Pastan: Dr. Gill's question I think was directed toward neuroblastoma cells?

G.N. Gill: I'll be glad to extend it to any of the cells lines discussed.

I. Pastan: There's been one publication by Gericke and coworkers who claim that treating animals with a lymphoma with cyclic AMP decreases the growth rate of the lymphoma. We have been engaged in following up on these studies by treating mice inoculated with polyoma transformed fibroblasts with dibutyryl cyclic AMP. Our results in general have been negative, i.e., lots of tumor growth, or no inhibition.

J. Roth, Yale University: I was wondering about your transport studies. You did time points at two hours, in the hour range. Was that the time intervals you were using?

M. Lubin: What was done, was to treat with cyclic AMP over a long period of time, but we would use a half hour pulse at each time point. This is important because if you simply add the radioactive material at the start of a 12 hour experiment, we found that incorporation may not be linear with time as you would normally hope. It depends on the amount of substrate you are adding and other changes, so these were experiments for defined intervals 4,8, and 12 hours.

J. Roth: The reason I ask is because I found in the transport of phenylalanine that the uptake of phenylalanine is linear only up to about 90 seconds; it's a very quick process. If you want to look at only the uptake of phenylalanine or some other metabolite, you would have to look at a time pulse of about a minute, samples taken every 15 seconds, because otherwise you would produce a host of other parameters such as the steady state equlibrium of the amino acid pool, of the nucleoside pool and the degradation and synthesis of the macromolecules from the lower weight metabolites.

259

M. Lubin: That's quite right. In our case, we were interested in the total number of counts that were in the cell, that were still capable of being incorporated into DNA. For example, if some of the deoxycytidine were converted into another product on the way to DNA synthesis, but still not incorporated, we would want to pick that up in the TCA soluble pool. I think both have to be done, short term and longer experiments.

G.Weber, Indiana University: Have you used theophylline in any of these experiments?

M. Lubin: Yes, not systematically, largely because we did not see any profound enhancement of the effects of dibutyryl cyclic AMP.

G. Weber: More specifically, in the experiments where you found an interference with the uptake of thymidine, have you used theophylline?

M. Lubin: No, not in the experiments that we showed. Do you have a particular reason for asking?

G. Weber: Yes, I do, because we find that theophylline competitively inhibits the uptake of thymidine in liver slices and tumor slices. This is preliminary data. This is my interest in your presentation.

C. Tihon, St. Louis University: I have a few questions about your agglutination experiments and the virus content of the cells. Have you ever tested for reverse transcriptase activity?

M. Lubin: To see whether or not after dibutyryl cyclic AMP there might be an increase or decrease in reverse transcriptase, for example? We have not done that.

C. Tihon: With the agglutination experiments. I think both Dr. Prasad, and you showed the results in numerical forms like 3,4,4+ and I didn't see a dose effect of concanavalin A for example, from 20 micrograms or 50 micrograms to 500 micrograms per ml. Or perhaps you didn't see any change? I don't know whether you and Dr. Prasad are doing the same type of con A experiments.

R.N. Prasad: The Con A concentration which we used was about 135 and 250 micrograms per million cells and that had been the usual dosage used with the fibroblasts.

C. Tihon: The reason I asked this is, with Chinese hamster ovary cells, I've shown that treatment with dibutyryl cyclic AMP, produces a fantastic increase of virus production, and along with this, the cells show tremendous increase of agglutinatability. If you are using high concentrations of Con A, it is difficult to tell the increase in agglutination, but when you lower the concentration of Con A, the difference will show up quite nicely.

M. Lubin: Dr. Furmanski always did a range of concentrations, but I think our experiments are defective for simply looking for viruses because I think your implication's quite right. There are many ways to look for virus production, including reverse transcriptase, the use of BudR or IudR or other agents to induce viruses.

C. Tihon: The cloning efficiency of the cells are different, control cells at 62%, and the cyclic AMP treated cells at 14%. I wonder whether this would have an effect on the agglutination experiments.

M. Lubin: Although cloning efficiency was down, the cells were still intact and excluded trypan blue. In the agglutination assay, all cell numbers were adjusted to the same concentration. So I think not.

THE SYNTHESIS AND SECRETION OF COLLAGEN

P. BORNSTEIN, K. von der MARK,
H.P. EHRLICH and J.M. MONSON
Departments of Biochemistry and Medicine
University of Washington

Abstract: A biosynthetic precursor of collagen, procollagen, has been identified in cultures of fibroblasts and cranial bone. As obtained by acetic acid extraction, procollagen contains an additional sequence of some 200 amino acids at the NH_2-terminus of each of the three chains of the molecule. The amino acid composition of these sequences differs markedly from that of collagen. Antibodies to the proα chain specifically recognize determinants in this non-triple helical region and may prove useful in following the intracellular translocation of the protein by antibody labeling techniques at the electron microscope level.

When care was taken to prevent partial proteolysis during extraction, procollagen was shown to contain yet additional noncollagenous regions linked by disulfide bonds. A neutral proteolytic activity (procollagen peptidase) is capable of converting acid-extracted procollagen to collagen in vitro. Whether this reaction represents a step in the conversion of procollagen to collagen in vivo remains to be established.

Antimitotic agents retard the conversion of procollagen to collagen and inhibit the secretion of procollagen. Microtubules may therefore be involved in intracellular movement of the protein. A cytochalasin B-sensitive step has also been implicated in the secretory process.

These recently identified steps in the biosynthesis of a functional collagen molecule increase the potential for specific biochemical intervention in the process of collagen production.

263

INTRODUCTION

Cellular elements in solid tissues require an extra-cellular matrix and an intact blood supply for viability and growth. These requirements apply equally to many solid neoplasms; in the absence of a proliferating vascular supply, expansion of a tumor ceases due to the nutritional limitations imposed by diffusion (1).

Relatively little is known of the origin and nature of the desmoplastic response to neoplastic growth. It seems likely, however, that normal endothelial and connective-tissue-producing cells adjacent to a focus of a tumor are stimulated to provide a vascular supply and stroma favorable for growth of the neoplasm (2). Under such circumstances the ability to interfere with the synthesis and secretion of an important component of the matrix, such as collagen, may provide a useful means of controlling neoplastic growth.

In an attempt to better understand the process in-volved in collagen biosynthesis and to identify potenti-ally controllable steps, we have studied the cellular events which mediate the synthesis and secretion of this protein. The biogenesis of collagen possesses unusual features in that several unique post-translational modi-fications are required in order to transform the molec-.le into a structural subunit of a functional collagen fiber. These include the hydroxylation of peptidyl prolyl and lysyl residues (3) and the modification of lysyl and hydroxylysyl side chains leading to the formation of inter-chain covalent cross-links (4).

More recently it has become apparent that a precursor form of collagen, procollagen, exists (5-7). Procollagen may serve a number of functions including initiation of triple helix formation, transmembrane movement, and control of fiber formation. Efforts in our laboratory have been directed toward establishing the biochemical characteristics of the precursor and the subcellular processes involved in its cellular translocation and secretion, and in defining the manner in which conversion of procollagen to collagen occurs.

EXPERIMENTAL

Isotopically labeled procollagen was prepared by incubation of cranial bones from newborn rats or day 17 chick embryos in a modified Dulbecco's Eagle's medium in the presence of [2,3^{3}H]proline, [^{35}S]cysteine, or [G-^{3}H]tryptophan (5,8). The isolation of procollagen by acetic acid extraction and fractionation of the protein into its constituent proα chains by CM-cellulose and molecular sieve chromatography have been described (8,9). Purified proα1 chains were cleaved with CNBr and collagenase, and a fragment containing the sequence unique to the precursor chain was isolated by ion-exchange and molecular sieve chromatography (9). Procollagen was also extracted from bone with 1 M NaCl or 8 M urea at neutral pH in the presence of N-ethyl maleimide (NEM), diisopropylfluorophosphate (DFP) and EDTA (10).

Procollagen peptidase was prepared by homogenization and extraction of chick embryo cranial bones in 0.05 M Tris-HCl, pH 7.5, containing 0.15 M NaCl and 5 x 10^{-3} M CaCl$_2$ (11). The extract was centrifuged at 100,000 x g and the supernatant concentrated by pressure filtration. Protein precipitating between 15% and 50% saturated (NH$_4$)$_2$SO$_4$ was redissolved in the extraction buffer and constituted the enzymatic activity.

Isolated cranial bones were incubated in the presence of [^{3}H]proline and colchicine (1 x 10^{-4} to 3 x 10^{-6} M), vinblastine (5 x 10^{-5} M) or cytochalasin B (2.25 or 5 μg/ml). The extent of conversion of procollagen to collagen was assayed by determination of the relative proportions of isotopically labeled proα1 and α1 chains in the extracted protein by CM-cellulose chromatography (12). The radioactivity in the combined proα1 and α1 peaks provided a measure of total procollagen (and collagen) synthesis.

Rabbits were immunized with repeated injections of 0.2 mg of chick bone proα1 in complete Freund's adjuvant. Antibodies of proα1 were detected by a sensitive radioimmunoassay (13) which employed radiolabeled chick proα1 chains and a sheep anti-rabbit γG globulin serum. The specificity of such antisera was determined by inhibition immunoassays using proα1 chains and CNBr and collagenase fragments containing a major fraction of the sequence unique to the pre-cursor chain (14).

Chick embryo tendon cells were isolated as described by Dehm and Prockop (15) and maintained in monolayer cultures in a medium containing 40% NCI, 45% Hanks salt solution, 10% horse serum and 5% embryo extract (P. Bornstein and L. Garnett, in preparation). Pulse-chase experiments with [³H] proline were performed in 1 x 10⁻⁶ M colchicine in the absence of serum and embryo extract.

RESULTS

When rat or chick cranial bones were pulse labeled for 18 min and the newly synthesized collagen extracted with 0.5 M acetic acid, the pattern of radioactivity eluted from CM-cellulose differed from the optical density pattern contri-buted by carrier extracellular collagen (Fig. 1). A promi-nent peak of radioactivity (proα1) preceded the position of elution of the α1 chain. Under these conditions of chroma-tography proα2 and α2 coelute (16).

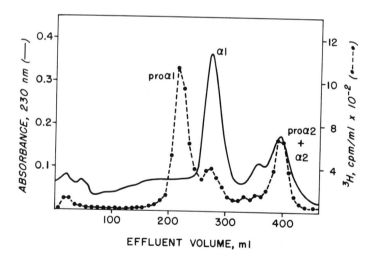

Fig. 1. CM-cellulose elution at 40° C of an acetic acid extract of chick cranial bones incubated with [³H]proline for 18 min. The sample was applied to the column in starting buffer, 0.04 M sodium

acetate, pH 4.8, in 4 M urea, and elution performed
by superimposition of a linear gradient of NaCl from
0 to 0.1 M over a volume of 700 ml. 10 mg of denatured
lathyritic rat skin collagen was added as an optical
density marker.

A molecular weight of 115,000 was determined for proα1
by calibrated molecular sieve chromatography and SDS gel
electrophoresis (8), in comparison with a value of 95,000
for α1. The amino acid composition of the additional
sequence in proα1 clearly differs from that of the α1 chain
(9) indicating that a region of the procollagen molecule
must exist in a conformation other than that of the collagen
triple helix. Initial studies by Uitto et al. (17) indicate
that the composition of the proα2 chain synthesized by chick
embryo fibroblasts resembles that of proα1.

In contrast to the pattern of elution of radioactivity
seen in Fig. 1, extraction of cranial bones with neutral
salt solutions in the presence of enzyme inhibitors yielded
an entirely different elution pattern (Fig. 2). The labeled
protein appears to be a disulfide-bonded procollagen since
reduction and alkylation produced proα chains similar to,
but larger than, proα chains obtained from acid-extracted
procollagen (10).

Evidence for a biosynthetic precursor role for procollagen was provided by pulse-chase experiments which
demonstrated a time-dependent conversion of procollagen to
collagen (5,10). A neutral proteolytic activity (procollagen peptidase) capable of converting acid-extracted
procollagen to collagen in vitro, has been identified in
extracts of cranial bone (11). The enzymatic activity was
irreversibly inhibited by acidic pH but was not affected by
DFP or by soybean trypsin inhibitor (11).

Additional properties of procollagen peptidase are summarized in Table 1. The activity of procollagen peptidase
was assayed by measurement of the extent to which the preparation converted a radiolabeled procollagen preparation to
collagen. A cumbersome but reliable index of this conversion was obtained by determination of the relative proportions of radioactive proα1 and α1 chains by CM-cellulose
chromatography. The data in Table I indicate that the enzy-

matic activity is inhibited by EDTA and that activity cannot be restored by replacement with Mg^{++}. Solutions of Ca^{++}, Mn^{++}, Zn^{++} and Cu^{++} were similarly ineffective in restoring activity. Procollagen peptidase was not inhibited by the sulfhydryl reagents NEM, cysteine or p-CMB, but activity was abolished by high concentrations of β-mercaptoethanol. A preliminary size fractionation by ultrafiltration indicated a molecular weight in excess of 100,000 for the enzymatic activity.

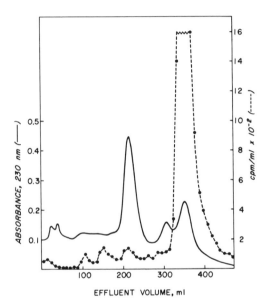

Fig. 2. CM-cellulose elution at 40° C of a neutral salt extract of chick cranial bones incubated with [^{3}H]proline for 18 min. See legend to Fig. 1 for additional details.

Thus far attempts to develop an assay for procollagen peptidase based on the ability of the enzyme to cleave synthetic substrates have not been successful. No demonstrable activity has been observed with 3-(2-furylacryloyl)-glycyl L-leucinamide (FAGLA), p-toluene sulfonyl L-arginine methyl ester (TAME) N-benzoyl L-tyrosine ethyl ester (BTEE), or with a synthetic pentapeptide used as a collagenase substrate.

TABLE 1

Properties of procollagen peptidase

Experiment	Recovery from CM-cellulose column (% cpm)	Proα1/α1
1 Buffer Control	64	2.33
Enzyme	72	0.66
Enzyme + 10 mM EDTA	81	2.90
Enzyme + 10 mM EDTA followed by dialysis against 5 mM MgCl$_2$	63	2.77
2 Buffer control	70	2.27
Enzyme	--	0.27
Enzyme + 10 mM NEM	79	0.52
3 Enzyme	85	0.37
Enzyme + 1 mM cysteine	71	0.34
Enzyme + 1 mM p-CMB	83	0.41
4 Enzyme	80	0.38
Enzyme + serum	79	0.58
5 Buffer control	70	1.91
Enzyme + 0.1 M 2-mercaptoethanol	77	1.86
6 Buffer control	50	1.23
<100,000 MW	59	1.28
>100,000 MW	60	0.57

It has not been possible to inhibit procollagen peptidase in organ cultures without inhibiting collagen synthesis as well. However, during the course of experiments designed to increase the yield of procollagen for structural studies, it was observed that compounds or agents which interfere with microtubule function retard the rate at which procollagen is converted to collagen. The most effective agents were the antimitotic compounds, colchicine and vinblastine (12, Table 2). Concentrations of colchicine as low as 1 μM were effective. These compounds did not inhibit non-collagen protein synthesis in short term incubations nor was the hydroxylation of the newly synthesized collagen affected. In contrast α,α' dipyridyl, an iron chelator which inhibits collagen proline hydroxylase, retarded conversion of procollagen to collagen (18, Table 2) but also markedly inhibited the hydroxylation of newly synthesized procollagen.

Deuterium oxide (100%), high hydrostatic pressure (10,000 psi), and uncouplers of oxidative phosphorylation also retarded the conversion of procollagen to collagen (12). None of these agents directly inhibited procollagen peptidase. It seems likely that microtubules translocate procollagen from its site of synthesis on polysomes to a site near the cell membrane. Thereafter the precursor is converted to collagen by limited proteolysis either in vesicles subjacent to the cell membrane, on the membrane itself or extracellularly. The precise locus of action of procollagen peptidase is still unknown and indeed may differ depending on the nature of the tissue and the extracellular environment (see Discussion). It would appear that interference with microtubular function impedes access of the collagen precursor to procollagen peptidase or other enzymes involved in its conversion to collagen, presumably as a consequence of intracellular compartmentalization.

In contrast to antimitotic agents, cytochalasin B did not retard procollagen conversion (Table 2). However, collagen synthesis (but not non-collagen protein synthesis) was inhibited. If an inhibition of uptake of labeled proline used as an indicator of new collagen synthesis can be excluded, a membrane-associated event in collagen secretion may be implicated.

270

TABLE 2

Modification of conversion of procollagen to collagen as
detected by the ratio of proα1 to α1 in extracts of
cranial bones.

Agent	Labeling period, min.	Proα1/α1 Control	Proα1/α1 Exp.	Exp/ Control	Synthesis, % Control
Colchicine (10^{-4} M)	30	0.26	1.80	6.92	71
Vinblastine (10^{-5} M)	45	0.32	1.29	4.08	60
Cytochalasin B. (5 μg/ml)	30	0.63	0.33	0.52	55
α,α'dipyridyl (1.4 x 10^{-3} M)	60	0.14	0.52	3.71	31

Tissues such as bone do not lend themselves readily to
a biochemical dissection of intracellular versus extracellular events. However, inhibition of secretion of collagen
by vinblastine has clearly been shown by autoradiography at
the light microscope level (unpublished experiments). A
more direct demonstration of this effect can be made with
chick embryo fibroblasts in monolayer culture (Table 3).
In the presence of 1 μM colchicine there was a three-fold
reduction in labeled non-dialyzable hydroxyproline in the
medium. Incorporation of labeled proline into cellular
protein was only slightly reduced and cellular peptide-
bound hydroxyproline was increased, findings which are
consistent with an inhibition of secretion of collagen.

The abundance of extracellular collagen poses a serious
obstacle to both morphological and biochemical approaches
to studies of the dynamics of the small intracellular pool
of this protein. We have recently developed antibodies to

the proα1 chain of procollagen which may prove useful in
studies of the intracellular translocation and secretion of
the protein (14). As shown in Fig. 3 both the proα1 chain
and a CNBr fragment containing the predominant antigenic
determinants of the chain inhibit the ability of antibodies
to combine with the radiolabeled test antigen. The α1
chain, even in 10 to 100 fold molar excess, produced no
inhibition under the conditions of the assay. The more
effective inhibition by the fragment compared with the
intact chain may be due to the higher solubility of the
fragment under the conditions of the assay or to the
increased tendency of proα1 to aggregate in the presence of
the large amount of α1 chain used during preliminary
absorption of the antiserum.

TABLE 3

Colchicine inhibition of secretion of peptidyl
hydroxyproline by cultured fibroblasts

Experiment	Labeling period, min.	Cells (cpm/mg cell prot.)		Medium (cpm/mg cell prot.)
		$\frac{\text{Total}}{\text{x } 10^{-4}}$	$\frac{\text{Hyp}}{\text{x } 10^{-3}}$	$\frac{\text{Hyp}}{\text{x } 10^{-3}}$
Control	90	6.98	5.85	8.00
Colchicine (1 μM)	90	6.45	7.92	2.86
Control	120	12.7	6.07	22.2
Colchicine (1 μM)	120	10.8	7.40	6.40

DISCUSSION

Efforts to regulate collagen synthesis are of more than
theoretical interest. The control of clinically undesir-
able scar formation such as occurs frequently following lye
burns of the esophagus, during surgical repair of nerves or

tendons, or as a concomitant of cirrhosis of the liver, represents an important objective. It would not stretch the imagination unduly to suggest that an effective means of inhibiting stromal proliferation in a neoplasm might provide a feasible means of checking neoplastic growth. Attempts to reduce scarring during an inflammatory response have been made by administration, both systemically and locally, of compounds which interfere with the normal covalent cross-linking of collagen extracellularly (19). Studies using proline analogues to inhibit peptidyl proline hydroxylation and secretion of collagen (3) have also been performed.

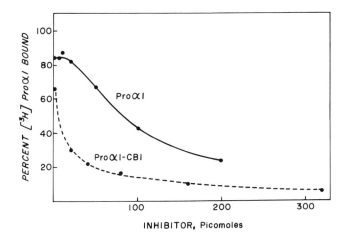

INHIBITOR, Picomoles

Fig. 3. Inhibition immunoassays with proα1 and proα1-CB1. The assay has been described in detail (13). 4000 cpm of ^{3}H-proα1 (about 10 picomoles) was used as a test antigen and 50 μl of a 1:5 dilution of a rabbit anti-proα1 serum as a source of antibody. 100 μg of α1 (1 nanomole) produced no inhibition. All determinations were performed in duplicate.

We have been concerned with an elucidation of the very complex process which leads from the synthesis of a nascent polypeptide to the secretion of a functional triple-helical collagen monomer. The demonstration that collagen chains are synthesized as higher molecular weight precursors (5-7)

273

is important for many reasons, but in the context of this discussion because it establishes a requirement for a limited proteolysis step in the conversion of procollagen to collagen. Control of the appropriate proteolytic activity might provide a means of selectively affecting collagen synthesis and/or function. That collagen synthesis persists despite a deficiency of procollagen peptidase is suggested by experience with an inborn metabolic disorder of cattle, dermatosparaxis (20) in which a deficient activity of the enzyme has been identified (21). Animals with the disorder synthesize normal amounts of collagen but display severe dysfunction in tissues such as skin due to improper fiber formation. If the entire process of conversion of procollagen to collagen occurred extracellularly, synthesis and secretion of the precursor might not be affected by a lack of the enzymatic activity.

There is recent evidence, however, that the procollagen molecule obtained from acid extracts of bone represents only a derivative of the native precursor (10,22,23). Apparently a loss of disulfide-bonded sequences from the precursor may occur due to limited proteolysis by tissue enzymes. Conceivably, more than one proteolytic step may be involved in the conversion of procollagen to collagen and the initial cleavage may occur intracellularly (24). Different enzymes may be involved and the possibility exists that these enzymes, in turn, have precursor forms. Such a highly complex system for "activation" would not be unreasonable for modulation of a highly important cellular activity such as collagen synthesis and expands the scope for potential biochemical intervention (as well as the likelihood that a variety of different genetic disorders involving this pathway exist).

The role of microtubules in collagen secretion has been documented both in this laboratory and in others (25,26). Other subcellular structures may also be involved in the secretory process (27). However, similar mechanisms function in the intracellular translocation and secretion of a variety of extracellular proteins and hormones (27). Thus even though interference with microtubular function results not only in inhibition of secretion but also in diminished synthesis of collagen (12), the effect is not likely to be sufficiently specific to be useful.

A more promising approach to the control of collagen synthesis concerns the mechanisms by which fibroblasts are stimulated to synthesize and secrete the protein. It seems clear that the rapid elaboration of an extracellular matrix by previously quiescent cells occurs under a variety of circumstances, of which a rapidly growing neoplasm is only one. A number of possibly different chemical factors could interact with membrane-associated receptors leading to an enhancement of collagen synthesis. Naturally, one asks whether cyclic AMP is involved in the intracellular limb of this effect. The profound changes which occur in Chinese hamster ovary cells treated with cyclic AMP include a marked increase in collagen synthesis (28). An effect of cyclic AMP on collagen synthesis in normal fibroblasts is less clearcut but a stimulation has been reported (12,25). This matter is under further investigation.

It would be of considerable interest to identify and characterize membrane-associated structures which respond to extracellular chemical messages related to collagen production. We anticipate that antibodies to procollagen when labeled directly or indirectly with ferritin (29) will be useful in delineating the intracellular pathway for secretion of the precursor. Conceivably procollagen or a derivative thereof, functions in association with a membrane receptor involved in feedback inhibition of synthesis. If so, antibody labeling techniques at the electron microscope level may be useful in its localization on the cell membrane.

REFERENCES

(1) J. Folkman, E. Merler, C. Abernathy and G. Williams, J. Exp. Med. 133 (1971) 275.

(2) T. Cavallo, R. Sade, J. Folkman and R.S. Cotran, J. Cell Biol. 54 (1972) 408.

(3) M.E. Grant and D.J. Prockop, New Eng. J. Med. 286 (1972) 242.

(4) P.M. Gallop, O.O. Blumenfeld and S. Seifter, Ann. Rev. Biochem. 41 (1972) 617.

(5) G. Bellamy and P. Bornstein, Proc. Nat. Acad. Sci. USA 68 (1971) 1138.

(6) D.L. Layman, E.B. McGoodwin and G.R. Martin, Proc. Nat. Acad. Sci. USA 68 (1971) 454.

(7) P. Dehm, S.A. Jimenez, B.R. Olsen and D.J. Prockop, Proc. Nat. Acad. Sci. USA 69 (1972) 60.

(8) P. Bornstein, K. von der Mark, A.W. Wyke, H.P. Ehrlich and J.M. Monson, J. Biol. Chem. 247 (1972) 2808.

(9) K. von der Mark and P. Bornstein, J. Biol. Chem., in press.

(10) J.M. Monson and P. Bornstein, submitted for publication.

(11) P. Bornstein, H.P. Ehrlich and A.W. Wyke, Science 175 (1972) 544.

(12) H.P. Ehrlich and P. Bornstein, Nature New Biol., 238 (1972) 257.

(13) H. Lindsley, M. Mannik and P. Bornstein, J. Exp. Med. 133 (1971) 1309.

(14) K. von der Mark, E.M. Click and P. Bornstein, submitted for publication.

(15) P. Dehm and D.J. Prockop, Biochim. Biophys. Acta 240 (1971) 358.

(16) H.P. Ehrlich and P. Bornstein, Biochem. Biophys. Res. Commun. 46 (1972) 1750.

(17) J. Uitto, S.A. Jimenez, P. Dehm and D.J. Prockop, Biochim. Biophys. Acta 278 (1972) 198.

(18) P.K. Muller, E. McGoodwin and G.R. Martin, Biochem. Biophys. Res. Commun. 44 (1971) 110.

(19) P. Bornstein, in: Diseases of Metabolism, 7th Edition, ed. P.K. Bondy (Saunders, Philadelphia, 1973) in press.

(20) A. Lenaers, M. Ansay, B.V. Nusgens and C.M. Lapière, Eur. J. Biochem. 23 (1971) 533.

(21) C.M. Lapière, A. Lenaers and L.D. Kohn, Proc. Nat. Acad. Sci. USA 68 (1971) 3054.

(22) R.E. Burgeson, A.W. Wyke and J.H. Fessler, Biochem. Biophys. Res. Commun. 48 (1972) 892.

(23) B.D. Smith, P.H. Byers and G.R. Martin, Proc. Nat. Acad. Sci. USA 69 (1972) 3260.

(24) A. Veis, J.R. Anesey, J.E. Garvin and M.T. Dimuzio, Biochem. Biophys. Res. Commun. 48 (1972) 1404.

(25) P. Dehm and D.J. Prockop, Biochim. Biophys. Acta 264 (1972) 375.

(26) R.F. Diegelmann and B. Peterkofsky, Proc. Nat. Acad. Sci. USA 69 (1972) 892.

(27) P. Bornstein and H.P. Ehrlich, in: Biology of the Fibroblast, ed. E. Kulonen (Academic Press, London, 1973) in press.

(28) A.W. Hsie, C. Jones and T.T. Puck, Proc. Nat. Acad. Sci. USA 68 (1971) 1648.

(29) J.P. Kraehenbuhl and J.D. Jamieson, Proc. Nat. Acad. Sci. USA 69 (1972) 1771.

This work is supported by NIH grants AM-11248, DE-02600 and HD-04872. P.B. is the recipient of Research Career Development Award K4-AM-42582 from the U.S. Public Health Service. K. v.d.M. is supported by a NATO fellowship, H.P.E. by Training Grant AM-1000 and J.M.M. by Training Grant GM-00052. We thank C.C. Clark, E.M. Click, F. Arguelles and D. Wright for assistance.

DISCUSSION

A. Hsie, Oak Ridge National Laboratories: I just want
to contribute a piece of information for the purpose or recall. You comment that we had a very significant high increase of collagen synthesis in the system we studied, and
you don't find this increase. I want to mention that, because
of limitation of the space available in the publication, we
did not mention specifically the CHO cell line we used in
the control experiment. It only makes a very limited detectable amount of collagen. The only mention in the paper
is that it does have a significant increase. The increase
is of an amount still very low compared to levels found when
you use a high collagen producer. I want to comment on
the manuscripts, since we haven't published it for over
two years. We were able to show, and I think Dr. Puck
may wish to elude this point in his presentation this afternoon,
that we do find increases: this experiment was done in
collaboration with Dr. Keith Porter and Dr. Puck. What
Keith Porter found was there was a definite increase of
amount of microtubules per cell after cyclic AMP treatment.
They also had a definite change of the microtubule orientation
along the long axis of the cell, and this is in conjuction
with the collagen increase.

P. Bornstein, University of Washington: Thank you
for those comments. I was aware of the fact that this line
made only a very small amount of collagen. Clearly the
tissues and cells that we've been looking at are making
a great deal of the protein and one might not expect to see
quite the same effects on addition of cyclic nucleotides.

A. Hsie: And right there we can make this record
clear and I might add one point: using the technique we've

been using, sometimes you can see no synthesis of the collagen at all in the control cell.

D.R. Robinson, Massachusetts General Hospital: I am not quite clear what method was used to rule out the possibility that colchicine and vinblastin might have had inhibitory effects on the procollagen peptidase. I think you may have mentioned that peptidase levels were unchanged, but has the possibility been eliminated that there may be, in a test tube, an inhibitory effect of the peptidase activity on these agents added?

P. Bornstein: Those experiments were performed, and in fact, with the isolated enzymatic activity these agents did not affect the activity of the procollagen peptidase preparation.

C. Tihon, St. Louis University: Would you comment on the lability of the 5% hot TCA extraction method on the procollagen molecules since I understand that collagen can be extracted with 5% hot TCA.

P. Bornstein: Yes, collagen itself has the unusual property of being soluble in hot 5% TCA. It is not a very good way of extracting the protein because there is a significant amount of degradation of collagen by use of this method. We've not used it in any way in these experiments. I don't know how procollagen would behave in hot TCA.

C. Moore, Albert Einstein: In looking at some of the pictures that you had, I was reminded of two as normal situations. The first one is the hypertrophic scar, and the second one is the situation where some youngsters are born with a disease which results in hyperextensive skin. Can you tell me anything about the nature of the procollagen and the mature collagen under these conditions?

P. Bornstein: Well, your question raises the complex issue of how these findings relate to some of the clinical

problems that we see. It is very likely that a number of
the congenital abnormalities that have been identified, or
that are not well defined as clinical enities, may result
from one or another defect in this biosynthetic scheme.
There is a disorder of cattle that has been recently identified
by Charles Lapiere and his associates in Belgium called
dermatosparaxis, which seems to result from a defect in
procollagen peptidase, the enzymatic activity responsible
for the conversion of procollagen to collagen. These animals
have a variety of defects including a very friable skin,
to the extent that one can grasp the hide and tear if off
by hand. It is very likely that a number of disorders that
have been classified as Ehler's-Danlos syndrome will turn
out to have defects in conversion of the precursor procollagen
to collagen. With respect to hypertrophic scar, that is
likely to result from an imbalance in the synthesis and degradation of collagen during wound healing but the defect
is not well characterized.

C. Moore: There was an article that appeared in Proc.
Nat. Acad. Sci. in which a patient with hyperextensive
skin was described, and I think one of the enzymes involved
in the glycosylation must have been abberant. I was hoping
that you might be able to give a little more information about
this disease.

P. Bornstein: In that report, the patients had a defect
in collagen lysine hydroxylase; the hydroxylysine content
of the collagen was quite low. There appeared not to be,
as far as could be determined, a defect in the conversion
of procollagen to collagen. As a consequence of low
hydroxylysine content the intermolecular crosslinks that
normally stabilize the collagen fibers were defective. Apparently lysine cannot always replace hydroxylysine in the
formation of functional crosslinks, and it would appear
that the main problem in the two siblings described in that
paper was defective crosslinking resulting from inadequate
hydroxylysine synthesis.

A. Hsie: In the only experiment we have done with high collagen producing tissue culture cells, the effect of dibutyryl cyclic AMP is much less pronounced, but it does increase collagen synthesis. The magnitude of the increase is much less.

GENETIC BIOCHEMICAL STUDIES ON THE MAMMALIAN CELL SURFACE

THEODORE T. PUCK
Department of Biophysics and Genetics
University of Colorado Medical Center
Denver, Colorado

Abstract: The application of the methodologies of somatic cell genetics and genetic biochemistry has made it possible to ask many new questions about cell surface phenomena and the influence of various agents on cell behavior. It appears reasonable to hope that such studies may shed important light on the nature of cancer.

I. Introduction

A new approach to the study of the genetics of mammals was opened up by the use of somatic cells instead of the germ cells for genetic and microbiological studies. The methods of microbial genetics have been applied to somatic mammalian cells for purposes of clone production, quantitation of growth, mutant isolation, mutation induction, study of chromosomal constitution and variation, complementation analysis, gene ploidy analysis, dominance and recessiveness determination, reversion analysis of mutants, linkage determination, association of linkage groups with chromosomes, identification of control genes and biochemical identification of mutational blocks. These tools now also give promise of being useful in the study of differentiation processes. The present paper contains experiments dealing with cell surface phenomena and their implications for cancer. The experiments here summarized have been carried out by the following coworkers: Abraham Hsie, Carol Jones, Fa-Ten Kao, A. J. Kauvar, Ryushi Nozawa, David Patterson, Keith Porter, Theodore T. Puck, Carol Smith, Charles Waldren and Leonor Wenger. It is noteworthy that a number of our results on dibutyryl cyclic AMP were published simultaneously with similar ones from Dr. Pastan's laboratory, and the two laboratories have often corroborated, and complemented each other's findings, as well as each producing unique discoveries.

II.   The morphological states of the Chinese hamster
ovary cell CHO-Kl <u>in vitro</u>.   Tissue culture cells commonly
adopt one of two extreme modalities with occasional intermediate morphological forms.   This phenomenon is of particular interest in the transformation of benign cells to
the malignant state by means of carcinogenic, physical,
chemical or viral agents.   The change in morphology associated with such a malignant transformation can be produced
although in a reversed direction, by treatment of CHO-Kl
cells with dibutyryl cyclic AMP (Fig. 1).

(A)

(B)

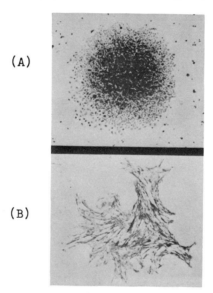

Fig. 1.   Effect of dibutyryl cyclic AMP (DBcAMP) on
the morphology of Chinese hamster ovary cells.   A, colony
grown from a single CHO cell on standard medium for 6 days;
B, colony grown in the presence of $10^{-3}M$ DBcAMP.

Cells originally in an epithelial status resembling that
of transformed cells change to a fibroblast-like structure and continue to multiply in a pattern like that of
the normal cell (Fig. 2).

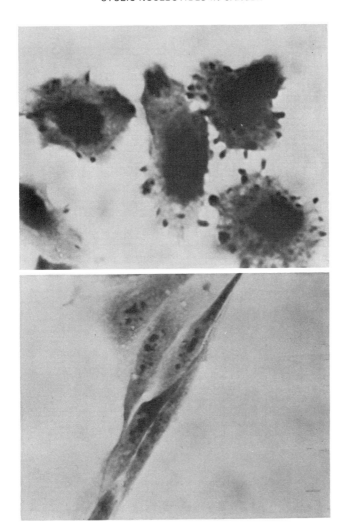

Fig. 2. Demonstration of the presence of knob-like structures in CHO cells grown for 18 hrs. in basal medium (above), and the disappearance of these bodies in a similar culture to which DBcAMP and testosterone was added (below). X1400

A list of the properties associated with the epithelial-like and the fibroblast-like morphologies, respectively, is shown in Table 1.

285

Table 1

Characteristics of the two morphological types of the CHO-K1 cells, produced by application or withdrawal of 10^{-3}M dibutyryl cyclic AMP (DBcAMP).

	Epithelial-like (E form) $\xleftrightarrow[\text{DBcAMP withdrawn}]{\text{DBcAMP added}}$	Fibroblast-like (F form)
a)	Compact, multipolar	Stretched, spindle-shaped.
b)	Knobbed	Smooth-surfaced except for occasional knobs at the ends.
c)	Knobbed regions of membrane are violently oscillating.	Surface movement limited to a relatively slow ruffling.
d)	Cells grow randomly without associating or orienting themselves.	Cells associate and lie parallel to their long axis. Cells also orient along scratches in the attachment surface.

(continued on next page)

Table 1 (cont.)

e)	Cells spontaneously detach from growth surface.	Cells more firmly adherent to growth surface and to each other.
f)	High binding capacity for lectins.	Low binding capacity for lectins.
g)	Low synthesis of collagen.	Definite collagen synthesis.

287

The changes produced by use of 10^{-3}M dibutyryl cyclic AMP (DBcAMP) are manifest within a few minutes at 37°. Smaller concentrations of the drug produce a less marked effect and require more time for their manifestation.

Two important differences between the change in morphology produced by the removal of dibutyryl cyclic AMP from a situation like that in Figure 1B and that which is produced by the use of a carcinogenic agent are a) in the former case, virtually 100% of the cells of a culture undergo the change, whereas with the use of carcinogenic agents only a fraction of the original population is so affected. b) moreover, the change produced by DBcAMP is completely reversible, whereas that produced by carcinogenic agents is irreversible. These characteristics make the changes produced by DBcAMP more readily quantitated, and subject to biochemical analysis but they also make more difficult the study of changes in malignancy associated with these changes in morphology. We call agents which cause the CHO-K1 cells to adopt the fibroblast-like habitus, F-agents or reverse transformation agents. It is obvious that these agents have produced important changes in the cell surface and possibly in other structures as well.

III. Other features of the action of F-agents on the CHO cells.
   A. The effect of cell density.
      When single, isolated cells are inoculated into petri dishes, their morphology is most strongly of the E type. As colonial growth progresses, some of the features of the E state are lost, presumably because of the cell-to-cell contact. The first of these to disappear is the knobs which are so characteristic of the E. state. Cells at the center of a dense colony may adopt the F-like form or intermediate forms even in the absence of transformation conditions. Apparently then, this action is an important feature of cell contact phenomena.
      B. Is the effect under study really due to cyclic AMP liberated inside the cell from the dibutyryl compound? Study of the cellular action of cyclic AMP is complex because of the existence of antagonistic enzymatic reactions which synthesize and degrade this

compound. The steady state at any time then, depends on the outcome of competing reactions some of which, at least, can operate with extremely high rapidity. Cyclic AMP alone, added to cells, is virtually without effect in this system. Theophylline, a specific inhibitor of phosphodiesterase activity in the cell, by itself produces a very small effect. The combination of cyclic AMP and theophylline, however, produces transition to the F state, in a fashion similar to that of the dibutyryl compound.

Of the two possible mono-substituted butyryl cyclic AMP's only the N-butyryl is active. This could mean that only the N-butyryl but not the O-butyryl compound is resistant to the action of the cellular phosphodiesterase.

C. Hormonal synergisms. Certain compounds, which by themselves are inactive or very weakly active in producing the F-transformation of CHO-Kl cells, can reduce by a factor of 10 or more the concentration of DBcAMP needed to achieve pronounced effect. Prostaglandins E_1, E_2, A_1 or A_2 in concentrations of $6 \times 10^{-5}M$ behave in this way. Prostaglandin $F_{2\alpha}$ also is active but higher concentrations are required. Testosterone, its two immediate precursors, androstendione and 17α-hydroxyprogesterone, and its metabolic product 5α-dihydrotestosterone, also exert such synergistic action. This latter action is specific since other compounds in the steroid metabolic pathways like cholesterol, hydrocortisone and 17β-estradiol are without any synergizing action (Fig. 3).

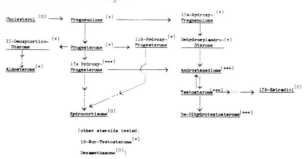

Specificity of steroids in producing conversion of CHO-Kl cells to a fibroblastic morphology when tested in the presence of 10^{-4}M (But)$_2$cAMP.

Fig. 3. Activity of various steroids in producing conversion of CHO-Kl cells to a fibroblast-like morphology when tested in the presence of 0.1mM DBcAMP. (+++), high activity; (+), some activity; (0), no activity. The diagram is arranged to show the biosynthetic relationship of the steroids.

Of particular importance as an experimental tool is the compound testololactone (Fig. 4), a microbial transformation product of testosterone.

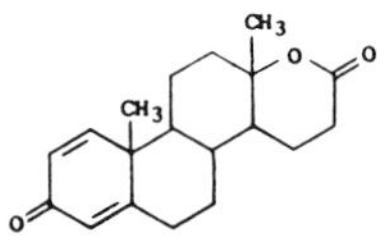

Fig. 4. Structure of testololactone

Testololactone was found to be much less inhibitory to growth than testosterone, but to exert its synergistic action in virtually the same concentrations as testosterone. Thus, maximal effectiveness of testololactone in aiding the conversion to the F state is achieved in concentrations between 5 and 10 µg/ml whereas compound does not inhibit growth materially until concentrations beyond 20 µg/ml are used.

D. Hormonal antagonism. Specific antagonism of the action of DBcAMP is afforded by the female hormone estradiol whose action, like that of the other materials studied, is reversible.

E. The effect of F-conditions on cell multiplication - growth in suspension and growth on plastic surfaces. The possible relationships of these effects to cancer make the question of growth promotion and inhibition of particular importance. While the phenomenon of contact inhibition of cell growth attached to glass or plastic surfaces has been taken as an index of the lack of malignant properties, the phenomenon itself is complex and appears to be influenced by a number of conditions which make difficult its careful study. We undertook study of a possibly more reproducible index, ability of cells to grow indefinitely in suspension, a phenomenon which appears to have good correlation with the malignant state.

When single cells of CHO-Kl are deposited on plastic surfaces, a distinct growth inhibition is observed if 10^{-3}M DBcAMP is used to achieve the fibroblast-like condition. However, if the F condition is achieved by means of 10^{-4}M DBcAMP plus 8γ/ml of testololactone, the toxic level of neither compound is reached and multiplication proceeds at the same rate as in the basal medium where E cells are produced. This would appear to be an important observation because it represents a change in differentiation state which is not necessarily related to a change in cell multiplication rate.

A very different situation occurs in the case of growth in suspension. The CHO-Kl cell resembles malignant cells in its ability to grow indefinitely at a high rate in liquid suspension cultures. The addition to such cultures of the standard DBcAMP testololactone mixture causes cessation of growth. This result suggests that the agents producing F morphology can maintain cell growth on surfaces but eliminates growth in suspension which is a characteristic of malignant cells.

IV. Provisional mechanism. Experiments with specific inhibitors have demonstrated that neither protein nor RNA synthesis is required for intraconversion of either

E or F cells into their respective opposite form. Apparently then the nature of these morphological conversions involves macromolecules already present in the cell which perhaps need only be organized in a new form.

The morphological change involved in conversion of E cells to the F type suggests an involvement of linear elements like the microtubules and the microfibrils. This possibility was supported by experiments that showed that passage from E into the F state could be prevented or reversed by the addition either of colcemide or similar agents which disorganize microtubules, or by cytochalasin B, which has been reported to disorganize the microfibrils.

A further experimental test of this hypothesis was carried out with the aid of Dr. Keith Porter in which cells prepared in the E and F states respectively were critically examined in the electron microscope. In these sectioned preparations, the number of microtubules per μ^3 of cytoplasm and the parallelism of their orientation were determined. These studies revealed a greater number of formed microtubules in the F form of the cell as compared with the E form. Of even greater interest, however, was the fact that the microtubules in the F form of the cell were organized in tightly packed parallel layers whose axis coincided with the long axis of the spindle-shaped cell. In contrast, those microtubules in the E form cells tended to be randomly oriented. The conclusion then seems well established that treatment with dibutyryl cyclic AMP and testosterone results in organization of the microtubules into parallel arrays.

Scanning electronmicroscopy was used to delineate the morphology of the knobs, which are present only in the E type cells. It revealed that the knobs are distinct from microvilli which have often been described on cell surfaces. The microvilli appear to remain unaffected by either forward or reverse transformation. The knobs disappear rapidly when reverse transformation agents are added. Examination of electron micrographs of sections through the knobs has shown them to have a high density of ribosomes.

Knob-like cell extrusions have been described in a variety of cells as a result of different kinds of treatments. Some of these appear to be a response to generalized toxicity. In order to establish the specificity of the knob-like structures described here, F type cells were exposed to a variety of toxic conditions including those produced by agents like fluorophenylalanine, pactamycin, actinomycin D, fluorouracil and actidione. None of these toxic situations produced knobs like those which occur spontaneously in CHO-K1 cells in the basal medium or when the F type cell is treated with cytochalasin B or colcemide. It seems reasonable then to infer that these knobs are a characteristic feature of the E state of the cell.

As a working hypothesis we have proposed that a sufficient quantity of cyclic AMP inside a cell causes polymerization of tubulin and parallel organization of a microtubular-microfibrillar system so as to cause elongation of the cell with a resulting spindle-like shape. These parallel structural elements are probably attached to the cell membrane at two points which represent the ends of the spindle. (The presence of these two unique attachment regions for the microtubules on the cell membrane is reminiscent of the situation which obtains in anaphase, when the microtubular system is anchored at two opposite ends of the cell membrane).

Randomization of the linear system of microtubules which occurs when the process is reversed produces a multipolar compact cell of the E type. The knobs might conceivably represent the empty attachment sites on the cell membrane for the microtubular-microfibrillar system. It is of interest in this connection that when reverse transformation agents are added to CHO-K1 cells the first observed phenomenon is the disappearance of the knobs and thereafter the cells begin the elongation process. It remains to be determined how these structural changes are associated with the altered biochemical and growth behavior of the cell, i.e. is organization of the microfibrils a necessary concomitant of enzyme induction, or do both phenomena originate from a common metabolic cause.

V. Studies on other types of cells. This undoubtedly oversimplified scheme would appear to afford a possible explanation for the wide range of morphologies of mammalian cells grown on surfaces in tissue culture. The actual level of cyclic AMP in cells would depend on exogenous supply of this material or its precursors, its rate of synthesis in the cell, and the activity of degrading enzymes. The effectiveness of the cyclic AMP in producing the organized state of the microtubular-microfibrillar system would also depend on the presence of synergizing and antagonizing molecules. Some simple predictions emerge from these considerations. One would expect that the addition of either colcemide or cytochalasin B to cells which are normally fibroblast-like in basal medium, would cause loss of their bipolar character, increased compactness, and appearance of the characteristic knob-like structures. This prediction was fulfilled using the V-79, a Chinese hamster cell originally isolated from the lung which maintains a fibroblast-like morphology, which grows rapidly when attached to plastic surfaces, and which fails to grow in suspension culture. Similar results were found with the HeLa cell which ordinarily grows as a compact epithelial-like cell on surfaces but displays relatively few knobs in this condition. Addition of colcemide to surface cultures of the HeLa cells brings out a typical array of the knobbed structures. Addition of dibutyryl cyclic AMP and testosterone reverses this action in both of these latter cells (Fig. 5,6,7).

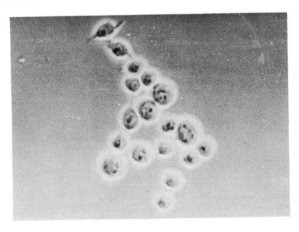

Fig. 5. HeLa cells grown in standard growth medium for 16 hours.

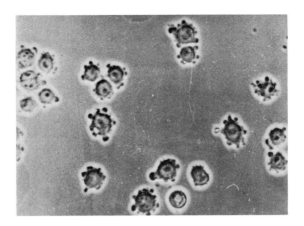

Fig. 6. HeLa cells identical to those of Fig. 5 to which 0.27 µM of colcemide was added and which were then incubated at 37° for 30 minutes. Note the resemblance between these knobbed cells and those of Fig. 2 (above). Since virtually all the cells of the culture are affected within 30 minutes by colcemide, the effect is not due to entrapment of cells in mitosis, but is a direct action of the drug on cells throughout interphase.

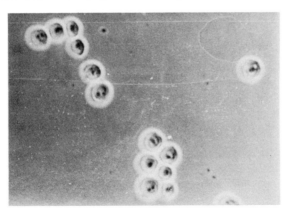

Fig. 7. HeLa cells identical to those of Fig. 5, but to which was then added a mixture of, 0.27 µM colcemide plus 1mM dibutyryl cAMP plus 15 µM testosterone. The reverse transformation conditions have completely prevented the production of knobs as in B. Cytochalasin B acts similarly to colcemide.

295

Continuing studies in this field involve the production and isolation of selected mutants and other variants with altered morphologies and altered susceptibilities to dibutyryl cyclic AMP, and the hormonal synergizing and antagonizing agents. Treatment of cells with mutagenic agents, selection of spontaneously occurring variants and the production of hybrids containing the Chinese hamster karyotype plus selected human chromosomes has now produced a variety of clones with variations in characteristics here discussed. These altered clones are being studied further (Fig. 8).

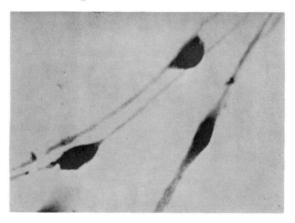

Fig. 8. A mutant clone of the CHO-K1 cell displaying an exaggerated response to the presence of DBcAMP and testosterone.

Experiments are also being conducted comparing the malignancy of these clones in the hamster cheek pouch.

VI. Methods for genetic study of specific surface antigens. The foregoing considerations make clear the importance of cell surface structure and behavior in determining vital areas of cellular metabolism which may be connected with differentiation and with cancerous properties. Work going on in many other laboratories, as for example that of Moscona and his coworkers, also has demonstrated the critical role played by cell surface

components. It became necessary, therefore, to attempt
to devise an approach which would facilitate genetic-
biochemical study of cell surface determinants.

Antibodies prepared against cells with specific
surface antigens can become lethal in the presence of
sufficient complement to permit lysis of the membrane in
the neighborhood of each specific antigen. Such lethal
surface antigens can be quantitatively and conveniently
detected by means of the single cell plating technique.
If human cells are hybridized with particular Chinese
hamster auxotrophs in appropriate selective media, one or
a few human chromosomes containing specific antigens can
be stably incorporated into a Chinese hamster cell.

Thus hybrids can be prepared containing different
specific human chromosomes and displaying different human
surface antigens. Antibodies prepared against the differentiated and undifferentiated human cells can then be
selectively adsorbed so as to leave the specific activity
against a single human surface antigen (Fig. 9).

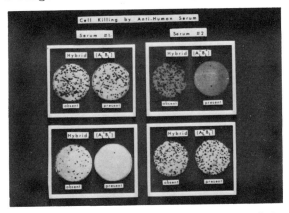

Fig. 9. Demonstration of the differential action of
A antiserum against A_L^+ and A_L^- cells; and of B antiserum
against B_L^+ and B_L^- cells.

Two different specific human antigens have been characterized in this way and have been named A_L, B_L. Hybrid cells
which are $A_L^+ B_L^+$, $A_L^+ B_L^-$, $A_L^- B_L^+$ and $A_L^- B_L^-$ have been

developed. Gene linkage can be readily determined for such markers by means of methodologies described in earlier papers. For example, the human A_L gene has been demonstrated to be linked to the lactic dehydrogenase A gene and not to the lactic dehydrogenase B gene (Fig. 10).

Tests for Linkage Between A_L and the LDH Isozymes, A and B.

Cell Phenotype	A_L: LDH-A:	+ +	+ -	- +	- -	A_L: LDH-B:	+ +	+ -	- +	- -
No. of clones found		41	0	0	35		24	17	9	26

Fig. 10. Demonstration of linkage between A_L and lactic dehydrogenase A, but not lactic dehydrogenase B.

This approach promises to make available new methodologies for study of the genetic determinants underlying the phenomena described in this paper.

REFERENCES

A. W. Hsie and T. T. Puck, Proc. Nat. Acad. Sci. 68 (1971) 358.
A. W. Hsie, C. Jones and T. T. Puck, Proc. Nat. Acad. Sci. 68 (1971) 1648.
F. T. Kao and T. T. Puck, J. Cell Physiol. 80 (1972) 41.
F. T. Kao and T. T. Puck, Proc. Nat. Acad. Sci. 69 (1972) 3273.
D. Patterson and C. A. Waldren, Biochem. Biophys. Res. Comm. (in press).
T. T. Puck, C. A. Waldren and A. W. Hsie, Proc. Nat. Acad. Sci. 69 (1972) 1943.
T. T. Puck, P. Wuthier, C. Jones and F. T. Kao, Proc. Nat. Acad. Sci. 68 (1971) 3102.

This investigation is a contribution from the Rosenhaus Laboratory of the Eleanor Roosevelt Institute for Cancer Research and the Department of Biophysics and Genetics (Number 529), and was aided by a U.S.P.H.S. Grant No. 5-P01 HD02080 and by an American Cancer Society Grant No. VC-81C. T.T.P. is an American Cancer Society Research Professor.

DISCUSSION

M. Chasin, Squibb Institute, Princeton: I would like
to comment on your steroid effect. Several years ago, our
group decided to investigate some compounds that are commonly used as drugs; included were about a hundred fifty
agents from some fifty therapeutic classes. This work was
recently published. It is of interest that of the steroids
we assayed, testosterone and testololactone were unique
in being inhibitors of cyclic AMP phosphodiesterase. I
suggest that this observation probably explains the potentiation
observed.

T. Puck, University of Colorado: This possibility
had occurred to us with these compounds. In our system,
the action of testololactone far exceeds anything we can
mimic with theophylline, so we have been cautious in
making interpretations. I am delighted to hear about your
results.

J.J. Voorhees, University of Michigan: Could you
describe how these changes with testosterone are different
from those that one would see with glucocorticoid? Dibutyryl
cyclic AMP mediated morphological changes in general
are due to post-translational modifications, and I understand
that you get synergism. I'm wondering if you have tried
to block the synergistic effect of testosterone by actinomycin
D?

T. Puck: In answer to your last question, the presence
of actinomycin D has no effect on the reverse transformation
produced by testololactone plus dibutyryl cyclic AMP.

J.J. Voorhees: And my first question had to do with
the addition of glucocorticoid to cells along with dibutyryl
cyclic AMP. Do you see an effect similar to that which
you observe with testosterone?

T. Puck: My memory is that nothing with the exception
of prostaglandins gave nearly as much effect as testosterone.

J. Kowal, University Hospital: What concentration
of colcemide and colchicine did you use in these experiments?

T. Puck: Approximately .02 micrograms per milliliter.

E.E. Smith, Boston University School of Medicine:
In view of present success of some workers to acquire poly -
merization of tubelin in vitro by means of low calcium,
I wonder if you have any opinion as to the role of calcium?

T. Puck: We've done a few experiments with ions that
suggest an effect of calcium, but these are too preliminary
to draw any conclusions, at this time.

J. Schultz, Papanicolaou Cancer Research Institute:
I want to apologize for introducing a quotation from the
New York Times, but it's the only source I have. Elliot
Osserman gave a talk at a dedication of the anniversary
of the discovery of lysozyme, and two large pictures were
shown: one of a spherical compact cancer-like cell,
and one of a very flat, apparently normal type of cell.
He stated that these were scanning electron micrographs
and that he accomplished that tranformation by the addition
of lysozyme. Did you by any chance have any experiences
of that type?

T. Puck: We have not carried out any experiments
with lysozyme.

K.N. Prasad, University of Colorado: Have you measured cyclic AMP levels in the clone which is spontaneously transformed to fibroblast like cells, and thus resemble dibutyryl cyclic AMP treated parent cells?

T. Puck: No, we have not done cyclic AMP levels in these cells.

G. Murison, University of Miami: I'm curious to know about the effects on the cell surface, that is, the ability to agglutinate with agglutinins. You mentioned that this is not effected by actinomycin. You see changes in the cell surfaces as reflected by the studies, do you also see changes in collagen production?

T. Puck: Yes, collagen of course is not produced in the presence of agents which inhibit synthesis. The binding of lectins has not yet been studied in the presence of inhibitors of protein synthesis.

G. Murison: What I'm trying to get at, is there any change in the distribution of ribosomes in the fibroblasts versus epithelial cells?

T. Puck: The only feature of which we can be certain so far is an unusually high concentration of ribosomes in the nobs which are present only in the epitheloid cells.

G. Murison: The question is not only the number of ribosomes, but there changes in their distributions, i.e., free vs. bound ribosomes, which might correlate with collagen production.

T. Puck: These are being looked at in the electron microscope the sections from which are now available.

ADENYL CYCLASE OF HUMAN SKIN AND ITS ABNOR-MALITIES IN PSORIASIS

S. L. HSIA, REBA K. WRIGHT
and KENNETH M. HALPRIN
Departments of Dermatology
and Biochemistry
University of Miami School of
Medicine

Abstract: After the incubation of slices of human skin with $[^3H]$ adenine in the presence of theophylline, ^3H was found in cyclic AMP, indicating the presence of adenyl cyclase in the skin. The accumulation of ^3H in cyclic AMP was enhanced by the addition of epinephrine or NaF in the incubation medium. Specimens from psoriatic lesions were significantly less effective in incorporating $[^3H]$ adenine into cyclic AMP, and the activity was less responsive to the stimulation of epi-nephrine and unresponsive to NaF, while the respon-ses of unaffected skin of the psoriatic patients to NaF and epinephrine were within normal range.

Adenyl cyclase activity was further demonstrated by the conversion of $[\alpha-^{32}P]$ ATP into cyclic $[^{32}P]$ AMP by homogenates of human skin. The enzyme was mainly associated with the 650 x g pellet, and respon-ded to the stimulation of epinephrine and NaF. The 650 x g pellet prepared from affected skin of psoriatic patients contained less adenyl cyclase activity than that prepared from the unaffected skin, and the acti-vity was not responsive to the stimulation of epi-nephrine and NaF.

Since psoriasis is characterized by epidermal hyperproliferation and accumulation of glycogen, the relevance of the observed abnormality of adenyl cy-clase to the disease mechanism deserves further investigation.

INTRODUCTION

Psoriasis is a scaly skin disease characterized by hyperproliferation of epidermal cells and the accumulation of glycogen in the lesion. Both these characteristics suggest there may possibly be a defect in a regulatory mechanism mediated by cyclic AMP. As the disease often affects large areas of the skin, it is possible to obtain strips of the diseased skin with a keratome for laboratory studies. This report deals with a comparative study of adenyl cyclase in skin specimens obtained from the affected and unaffected skin of psoriatic patients and from skin of control subjects. A preliminary report of this study was published previously (1).

EXPERIMENTAL AND RESULTS

1. Skin Specimens. Skin specimens were obtained with a keratome without anesthesia. The depth of the blade was set at 0.2 mm and micrographs of the cross section of these specimens showed that the cut was immediately below the basal cell layer in normal skin, while in the psoriatic plaque, some of the lowermost cells in the epidermal projections remained with the dermis. When the blade was set at 0.4 mm, the cut in psoriatic skin was under the basal cell layer. The specimens were divided into pieces of 30-50 mg, weighed on an analytical balance and immediately incubated as described below.

2. Incubation. The method of Kuo and De Renzo (2) for the study of adipose cells was adapated for incubation of the skin slices with $[^3H]$ adenine. The specimens (30-50 mg) were incubated at 37°C for 60 min with 5 μCi of ^3H adenine in 2 ml of Krebs-Ringer bicarbonate buffer at pH 7.4 under $O_2:CO_2$, 95:5 to label the ATP pool. The skin slices were then removed from the medium, rinsed with 0.9% saline, and incubated for another 30 min under $O_2:CO_2$, 95:5, in a fresh medium of 2 ml of

Krebs-Ringer bicarbonate buffer, pH 7.4, containing
10 mM theophylline, with or without NaF or epinephrine.

3. Isolation and Identification of $[^3H]$ Cyclic AMP.
The skin slices after the incubation were removed from
the incubation medium, rinsed with saline and boiled for
5 min in 1 ml of Tris buffer containing 1.25 μmoles of
cyclic AMP as internal standard for the determination of
the recovery of $[^3H]$ cyclic AMP, and 10 μmoles of theophylline for inhibition of the diesterase activity. The
boiled mixture was homogenized in a glass homogenizer
and centrifuged at 650 x g. The supernatant (0.5 ml)
was chromatographed on a column of Dowex AG 50W-X4
according to the procedure of Krishna et al. (3).

The fraction containing cyclic AMP was treated with
ZnSO4 and Ba(OH)2 to precipitate traces of ADP and
AMP. An aliquot of the solution was assayed for ^3H by
scintillation counting, and another aliquot was used for
the determination of recovery of cyclic AMP by measuring the absorbance at 259 nm.

The cyclic AMP fractions from several incubations
were pooled and subjected to thin layer chromatography
on polyethyleneimine impregnated cellulose using 0.6 M
ammonium formate as the developing solvent. The distribution of ^3H was determined by radioassay after
scraping the thin layer plate in sections. The result
showed a single peak of radioactivity corresponding to
the mobility of cyclic AMP (visualized by ultraviolet
light). The identification of $[^3H]$ cyclic AMP was further
substantiated by isotopic dilution and crystallization from
50% ethanol. The specific activity remained constant
after three crystallizations, and the result showed at
least 95% of the ^3H was in cyclic AMP.

4. Stimulation by Epinephrine and NaF. The effect of
epinephrine on the incorporation of $[^3H]$ adenine into
cyclic AMP is shown in Fig. 1. In separate experiments,

it was found that 1 to 2 µg of epinephrine per ml (approximately 5-10 µM) gave the maximum stimulation.

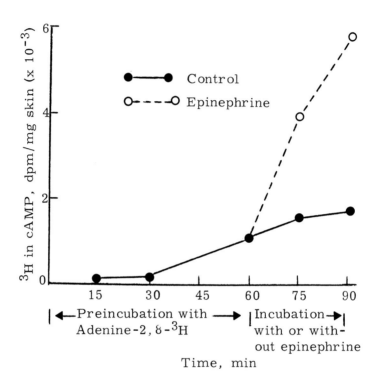

Fig. 1. Time course of incorporation of [³H]adenine into cyclic AMP by skin slices and the effect of epinephrine. After labeling the ATP pool by incubation with [³H]adenine, epinephrine (10 µM) was added to some of the incubations as indicated. (Data taken from reference (1)).

NaF also stimulated the incorporation of ³H adenine into cyclic AMP, and maximum stimulation was obtained at 10 mM NaF.

5. Comparison of psoriatic skin with unaffected skin of the patients and with skin of control subjects. The ability of skin slices to incorporate [3H] adenine into cyclic AMP was compared among three types of specimens: a) skin from 18 control subjects, b) psoriatic plaques from 11 patients, and c) unaffected skin from 5 of the psoriatic patients. The results are shown in Fig. 2.

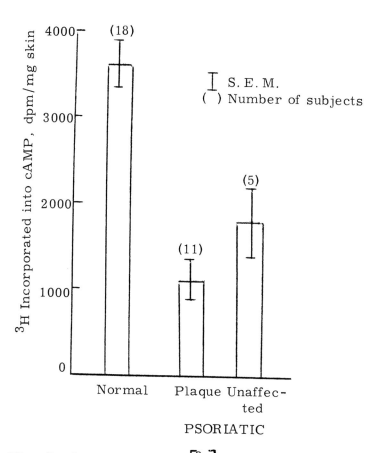

Fig. 2. Incorporation of [3H] adenine into cyclic AMP by normal skin, psoriatic plaque, and unaffected skin of psoriatic patients. The procedures for incubation and assay for [3H] cyclic AMP are described in the text.

The data show a considerable range of individual variations in each group. However, specimens taken from
the same individuals on different days gave results
varying within 10-15%.

The results from the psoriatic plaques were significantly lower than those from the controls ($p < 0.002$),
and did not overlap with results from the control group.
One specimen from the control group, however, had low
activity, and fell in the range of the psoriatic group.
The activity of the unaffected skin was higher than that of
the plaques ($p < 0.05$); this was the case in each of the
5 patients examined. Although the mean activity of the
unaffected skin was lower than that of normal skin, the
values overlapped. Because the number of specimens
examined was small, whether the unaffected skin had
normal activity or not was uncertain. The incubation
medium in each of the above experiments was examined
for $[^3H]$cyclic AMP after the incubation. The amount of
^3H in cyclic AMP was not detectable. The less than
normal amount of $[^3H]$cyclic AMP found in psoriatic
plaque after the incubation with $[^3H]$adenine was therefore not due to leakage of $[^3H]$cyclic AMP into the medium.

Since the psoriatic plaque is thicker than normal epidermis, for comparison, a 0.4 mm and a 0.2 mm specimen were obtained from the psoriatic plaques of one patient and incubated with $[^3H]$adenine. The result showed
that the 0.4 mm specimen had about half of the activity
of the 0.2 mm specimen. Thus the observed lower activity in psoriatic plaque was more exaggerated in the
thicker specimens which contained all the epidermal cells.

The response to NaF by the three types of skin is
compared in Fig. 3. It is significant that 10 mM NaF
had little or no effect on the psoriatic plaques, while
more than doubled the activity in normal skin and the
unaffected skin of the psoriatic patients.

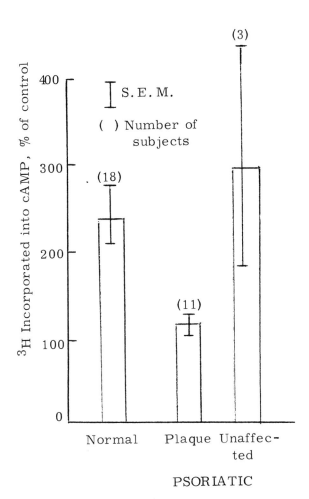

Fig. 3. Response to NaF by normal skin, psoriatic plaque and unaffected skin of psoriatic patients. The concentration of NaF in the incubation medium was 10 mM.

A comparison of the response to epinephrine by the three types of skin is shown in Fig. 4.

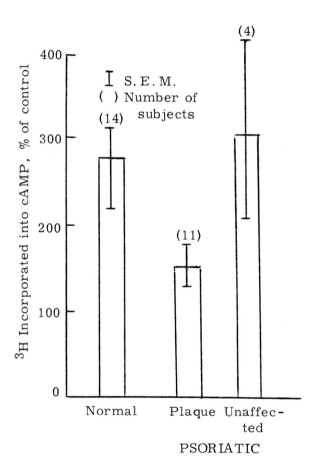

Fig. 4. The response to epinephrine by normal skin, psoriatic plaque and unaffected skin of psoriatic patients. The concentration of epinephrine in the incubation medium was 11 μM (2 μg/ml).

The response by the psoriatic plaques was significantly lower than by normal skin (p < 0.01). The unaffected skin seemed to have normal response.

310

These results suggested a possible defect in adenyl cyclase in psoriatic skin. But because the information obtainable by incubating skin slices with $[^3H]$ adenine was limited, we pursued the problem by another approach.

6. Broken-cell preparations. In addition to incubation of skin slices with $[^3H]$ adenine, we investigated adenyl cyclase activity in broken-cell preparations of the skin. To establish experimental conditions, skin specimens (0.2 mm thick) were obtained from a cadaver 4 hr post mortem, and ground in a glass tissue homogenizer at 0^oC in 8 volumes of 50 mM glycyl glycine buffer, pH 7.5, containing 8 mM $MgSO_4$ and 0.25 M sucrose. The homogenate was successively centrifuged at 4^oC at 650 x g for 15 min, 9700 x g for 30 min, and at 105,000 x g for 60 min. The pellets were washed twice with the homogenizing medium by resuspension and centrifugation. The homogenate, the washed pellets and the supernatants were assayed for adenyl cyclase activity by incubation with $[\alpha-^{32}P]$ ATP. The homogenate and each of the subcellular fractions, containing 0.5 mg of protein, were incubated at 30^oC for 10 min in 0.25 ml of 50 mM Tris buffer, pH 7.4, containing 20 mM theophylline, 8 mM $MgSO_4$, 0.25 mg bovine serum albumin, and 2 mM ATP labeled with 10^7 dpm of $[\alpha-^{32}P]$ ATP.

The incubation was terminated by the addition of 30 μmoles of ATP to dilute the labeled substrate, and 0.625 μmoles of cyclic AMP as internal standard for measuring the recovery of $[^{32}P]$ cyclic AMP. The mixture was boiled for 3 min, and the coagulated proteins were removed by centrifugation. The supernatant was chromatographed on Dowex AG 50W-X4, and the fraction containing cyclic AMP was assayed for ^{32}P by scintillation counting and the recovery of cyclic AMP by measuring absorbance at 259 nm.

The distribution of adenyl cyclase activity in the broken-cell preparation is shown in Table 1.

Table 1. Distribution of Adenyl Cyclase Activity in Human Skin

	Cyclic AMP Formed	
	pmoles/ min/g skin	pmoles/min/ mg protein
Homogenate	226	1.88
650 x g pellet	553	7.04
650 x g supernatant	80	2.47
9700 x g pellet	17	5.67
9700 x g supernatant	65	2.90
105,000 x g pellet	3	2.20
105,000 x g supernatant	50	0.65

The data show that the 650 x g pellet had the greatest amount of adenyl cyclase activity and also the highest specific enzymic activity. Further experiments with the 650 x g pellet showed that the enzyme had optimum activity between pH 7.5 and 8, and an apparent Km of 1 mM.

Adenyl cyclase activity in the 650 x g pellet was influenced by NaF, epinephrine, prostaglandin E_2 and other affectors. The results are shown in Table 2.

Table 2. Affectors of Adenyl Cyclase in the 650 x g Pellet of Human Skin

Additions	$[^{32}P]$ Cyclic AMP Formed	Percent of Control
	pmoles/min/mg protein	
Experiment 1		
None (control)	6.8 ± 0.7	100
Epinephrine, 4.5 μM	10.0 ± 1.10	148
Fluoride, 10 mM	13.8 ± 1.50	204
Insulin, 1 unit/ml	3.6 ± 0.1	53
Insulin, 1 unit/ml + epinephrine, 4.5 μM	5.8 ± 2.0	86
Experiment 2		
None (control)	7.4 ± 0.6	100
Epinephrine, 9 μM	11.7 ± 1.4	158
PGE$_2$, 44 μM	18.8 ± 1.3	254
Fluoride, 10 mM	18.3 ± 2.0	247
Propranolol, 10 μM	6.8 ± 0.7	92
Epinephrine, 9 μM + Propranolol, 10 μM	7.7 ± 0.8	104

The effects of epinephrine and NaF were further tested in a number of preparations from normal skin, and the results are shown in Fig. 5.

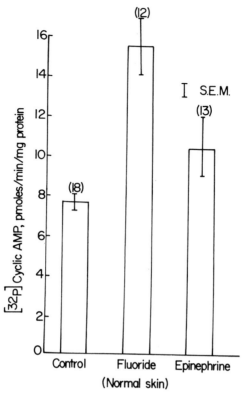

Fig. 5. Stimulation of adenyl cyclase activity by NaF and epinephrine in the 650 x g pellet of skin homogenates from control subjects. The concentration of epinephrine used was 11 μM, and the concentration of NaF was 10 mM

The average increase of activity in response to NaF was about 100%, and to epinephrine, about 40%.

The responses to epinephrine and NaF by the 650 x g pellets prepared from psoriatic plaques and unaffected skin of psoriatic patients are compared in Fig. 6. The preparations from the psoriatic plaque had less adenyl cyclase activity than that from normal skin ($p < 0.05$), and did not respond to NaF or epinephrine. Adenyl cyclase activity in preparations from unaffected skin and the responses to epinephrine and NaF were similar to those in normal skin, or slightly less than in normal skin. Because the number of specimens studied was small, the difference, if any, between normal skin and unaffected skin was not certain.

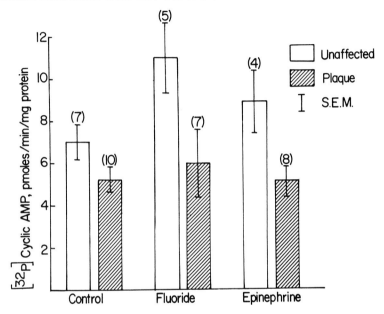

Fig. 6. Adenyl cyclase activity in psoriatic plaque and unaffected skin of psoriatic patients. The concentration of epinephrine used was 11 μM, and the concentration of NaF was 10 mM.

A time course of the formation of $[^{32}P]$ cyclic AMP from $[\alpha\text{-}^{32}P]$ ATP by the 650 x g pellets prepared from psoriatic plaques and unaffected skin of a patient is depicted in Fig. 7. The 650 x g pellet prepared from psoriatic plaques had about half the adenyl cyclase activity as in the preparation from unaffected skin.

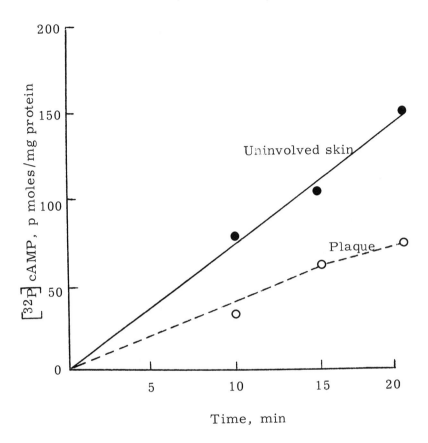

Fig. 7. Time course of formation of $\left[^{32}P\right]$ cyclic AMP.
The 650 x g pellets prepared from specimens of psoriatic plaque and unaffected skin of a psoriatic patient were
incubated with $\left[\alpha\text{-}^{32}P\right]$ ATP in the presence of 20 mM
theophylline. Each point is the mean of three determina-
tions. (Data taken from reference (1)).

Thus the results from experiments with the 650 x g
pellet corroborated findings in the experiments with skin
slices. The results from both types of skin preparations

suggested that the adenyl cyclase in psoriatic skin might be abnormal. In our limited number of observations, not only the enzymic activity seemed lower in psoriatic skin than in normal skin, but the responses to NaF and epinephrine also appeared defective, indicating that the enzyme in psoriatic skin may have defects at the receptor site(s) for the stimulators.

There are many inherent difficulties in working with the skin, and adenyl cyclase happens to be a difficult enzyme to assay. The number of patients willing to participate in such a study has also been small. The progress in this study is understandably slow. These results must be treated as preliminary data and need confirmation by a more extensive study.

In light of recent findings of Voorhees et al. (4) that the content of cyclic AMP in psoriatic skin is lower than in normal skin, defects in adenyl cyclase or in the control of its activity deserve attention.

REFERENCES

(1) S. L. Hsia, R. Wright, S. H. Mandy and K. M. Halprin. J. Invest. Derm. 59 (1972) 109.

(2) J. F. Kuo and E. C. De Renzo. J. Biol. Chem. 244 (1969) 2252.

(3) G. Krishna, B. Weiss and B. B. Brodie. J. Pharmacol. Exp. Ther. 163 (1968) 379.

(4) J. J. Voorhees, E. A. Duell, L. J. Bass and E. R. Harrell. Arch. Dermatol. 105 (1972) 695.

DISCUSSION

R.L. Anderson, Procter and Gamble, Co: Does the 650G precipitate have any phosphodiesterase activity?

S.L. Hsia, University of Miami: Yes, there is diesterase activity in the 650 x g pellet, but if you look into the distribution of the diesterase activity, you find this fraction contains much less diesterase activity than the supernatant from this fraction. Dr. Hurst is the one who did the work, maybe she wants to answer this question.

R.W. Hurst, University of Miami: The level of the phosphodiesterase activity in the pellet is higher than that of adenyl cyclase, but if you wash the 650G pellet several times you can decrease the phosphodiesterase activity until it's undetectable by our method of assay.

R.L. Anderson: Was a lot of the ^{32}P in 5'-AMP when you're using your 650G precipitate, in other words, have you inhibited the phosphodiesterase?

R.W. Hurst: We haven't measureed that, so I don't know how much ^{32}P 5'AMP is formed. We do include in these assays a phosphodiesterase inhibitor; we started out using theophylline, and then switched to papaverine. With 1 mM papaverine, we obtained 90% to 95% inhibition of phosphodiesterase activity.

R.L. Anderson: Thank you.

J.J. Voorhees, University of Michigan: Did you find it necessary to use an ATP regeneration system in your studies on psoriatic plaques?

S.L. Hsia: We did not find it necessary. We had some experiments using an ATP regenerating system, and the results were not different from those without using the regenerating system. We also measured the ATPase activity in the pellet and found the activity rather low.

J.J. Voorhees: That's very interesting because one of the things that we found early on our purified, very active membrane fractions from mammalian epidermis was that without an ATP regenerating system, we had most of our product in adenosine within 5 minutes. If you have practically no ATPase in the pellet, then would the possibility exist that you have a fair amount of dead membranes in that pellet, since ATPase would probably be very high in psoriatic epithelium? That was my first question. The second has to do with the sucrose density gradients. It struck me that your hormonally sensitive membrane fraction was floating. In other words, that your light membranes were high on the gradient and that your membranes that had less sensitivity were at the bottom of the gradient, indicating, as you know, that when epidermis differentiates the membranes get heavier. Therefore, if you are assaying the heavy membranes, they are more apt to be dead than alive, and that ought to concern you. Do you have any comments on that?

S.L. Hsia: In answer to your first question, I believe you're referring to your experiments using the 16,000 x g pellet, and we were using the 650 g pellet.

J.J. Voorhees: Right.

S.L. Hsia: We did use the 16,000 g pellet to repeat your work. We found the ATPase activity in that pellet much higher than in the 650 g pellet which we were using, so there was a difference in the selection of preparations of the membrane.

J.J. Voorhees: That would corroborate my concern, in other words, what we did was differential centrifugation and in the first, 650 g we took off the heavy stuff on the outside and in the electron microscope one can see that. You can see these very heavy looking membranes in stratum corneum, etc., with Hashimoto's dense band, etc. Then if you spin the 1,000 g supernatant at 17,000 g, that is where you find nice adenyl cyclase activity and that's where you just said you found the ATPase activity, is that correct?

S.L. Hsia: That's correct.

J.J. Voorhees: Seems to me that that's a pertinent point.

S.L. Hsia: Yes. I think that during the work, we are apt to disrupt these membranes, so that the lighter fraction of the membranes float on top. I just don't know where these low density membranes come from. They could very well come from the lower cell layer as well as from the top layer, because when you grind tissue and then subject to centrifugation at the end, you really don't know where this light fraction comes from. I don't believe that really represents membranes from cells in the higher layer. I don't believe that at all.

J.J. Voorhees: Would you agree that it's a possibility?

S.L. Hsia: Oh, I would keep all doors open to things like this. But the fact was that these lighter membranes did not respond to epinephrine while the heavier membranes did. This may mean the separation of the catalytic site from the regulatory site of the enzyme. There may be two sites on the enzyme and we are seeing their separation.

A.E. Lorincz, University of Alabama: Have you had no opportunity to look at other clinical conditions where you have epithelial proliferation?

S.L. Hsia: We have only very limited experience in looking at other skin conditions. We did examine a few specimens of Darier's Disease and atopic dermatosis. But I can't say much about the results, simply because we looked at just a few specimens. Again the problem is that of getting specimens.

R.A. Hickie, University of Saskatchewan, Canada: In one of your slides it looked as if insulin increased cyclic AMP formation. Was this statistically significant?

S.L. Hsia: I don't think it's statistically significant because we have done only one or two experiments. However, in experiments using skin slices and ^{3}H adenine, we have seen insulin blocking the stimulation of epinephrine rather than decreasing of the formation of cyclic AMP by insulin alone.

R.A. Hickie: Would you care to comment whether it's acting on the cyclase or phosphodiesterase?

S.L. Hsia: I don't think there is really good evidence one way or the other. Perhaps there is even another messenger system involved in insulin action. I don't think I can make any statement on how insulin affects the adenyl cyclase or the phosphodiesterase because we have no data base on which to speculate. Did you check the water difference in the tumor, or the placques versus normal skin? Is there any difference in water content?

K.M. Halprin, University of Miami: There's no difference in water content. They both contain two thirds water.

A. Hsie, Oak Ridge National Laboratory: Can an agent, or agents in combination, effectively elevate the cyclic AMP system and effectively cause the possible regression of psoriasis?

S.L. Hsia: Naturally, this is a question to which
everybody would like to find the answer. Many problems
are involved in testing something on a patient. You have
to have legal permission which we don't always have.
Besides, the permeability of many of the agents through
the epidermal barrier to get to the cell is a serious technical
problem.

P.A. Galand, Free University of Brussels, Belgium:
I have two questions dealing in fact with the same aspects
of your problems about the difference between levels in
cyclase activity. As you show clearly, the tissue in psoriasis
is very different, and mainly maybe it's different from the
viewpoint of the proportion of cells engaged in proliferative
activity as compared to cells not engaged in division.
Do you have any data on the incorporation of thymidine
into DNA as related to the total weight, or to the total
protein content of a given skin sample in normal skin
and in psoriasis? And the second question is another
approach to the same problem: did you try to find the
level of adenyl cyclase activity in fragments of tissue obtained
by consecutive stripping of skin samples in psoriasis and
normal skin?

S.L. Hsia: Well, I'll answer the last question first.
We have a time trying to obtain psoriatic specimens to
work with, leave alone various treatments. We therefore
have no information on stripped skin. In response to your
first problem about cell turnover, I believe Dr. Halprin
again can put some light on this subject.

K.M. Halprin, University of Miami: The only good
evidence on the cell turnover rate in psoriasis is by Dr.
Jerry Weinstein from our department. On a pro-rata basis,
I'm not sure those figures are so easily available, but the
data for the percent cells incorporating thymidine is available.
It's 3 to 5% in normal and 25% in psoriatic. The proliferative
pool in terms of layers of epidermal cells is probably about
$1\frac{1}{2}$ layers of normal epidermis and at least 3 layers of

proliferative cells in the psoriatic lesion. What proportion that is out of the total is kind of difficult to determine. I don't think there is really a large difference between the two. I would guess 1½ out of maybe 4 or 5 in normal, and 3 out of maybe 7 to 10 in the psoriatic layers of epidermal cells involved. I don't think there's a big difference in the two.

P.A. Galand: I knew these data from Weinstein's group, but in fact I think it would be interesting to try presenting your results as related to thymidine per milligram protein and see if the things are the same as when you put the results related to lipid metabolism as something else.

S.L. Hsia: Well, as I already mentioned, if you transpose the data from per milligram skin into per milligram protein, the difference between the psoriatic and the normal would be greater than what I've shown. If you express the results on the basis of DNA, it will be even more so.

S. Belman, New York University: What is the level of cyclic AMP in normal skin as compared to psoriatic skin?

S.L. Hsia: Dr. Voorhees will report this in the next paper.

G. Weber, Indiana University: I think we should keep in mind the remarkable discoveries of all these hormone actions, the rate of metabolic effects have played on the skin. Dr. Hsia explained to me the total weight of the skin is equal to that of the liver, so we have here an organ about the size of the liver which is reponsive in vitro to various hormones, and Dr. Hsia was able to establish cyclase activity, and phosphodiesterase activity. These studies are remarkable.

S.L. Hsia: Well, I might add that the weight of the skin really is even greater than that of the liver.

INCREASED CYCLIC GMP AND DECREASED CYCLIC AMP LEVELS IN THE RAPIDLY PROLIFERATING EPITHELIUM OF PSORIASIS

J. VOORHEES, W. KELSEY, M. STAWISKI,
E. SMITH, E. DUELL
Department of Dermatology
University of Michigan

M. HADDOX and N. GOLDBERG
Department of Pharmacology,
University of Minnesota

Abstract: Most common skin diseases, psoriasis being prototypic, accumulate glycogen in the presence of accelerated cell proliferation. This is paradoxical since it would seem that glycogenolysis should occur to fuel the proliferative process. We proposed that decreased cyclic adenosine monophosphate (cyclic AMP) levels could explain this paradox since the beta adrenergic inhibition of epithelial cell division is mediated by cyclic AMP as is glycogenolysis in liver and muscle. The measurement of cyclic AMP levels in involved epithelium versus uninvolved epithelium of the same 50 patients in comparison with that of 32 control subjects shows a highly significant decrease in the cyclic AMP levels of the lesion. Although experiments to elucidate the cause of this decrease are still in progress, at present we have not detected deficient cyclic AMP biosynthesis or excessive cyclic AMP hydrolysis.

Recently Goldberg and coworkers have shown that in a number of biological systems, elevated cellular cyclic GMP levels are associated with regulatory influences that oppose those promoted by agents that stimulate cyclic AMP generation. With regard to cell division and its control Hadden and Goldberg demonstrated increased cellular cyclic GMP accumulation in association with the induction of clonal proliferation of lymphocytes by mitogens. The latter suggested that elevated cyclic GMP levels might be associated with the depressed cellular concentration of cyclic AMP found in psoriasis. Upon measuring the levels of cyclic GMP in epithelium a highly significant increase in cyclic GMP concentration was found in the involved epithelium of psoriasis.

We wish to use this data, the concept of Tomkins and coworkers of pleiotypic control and Goldberg's theory of the "dualism" of biological control through opposing actions of cyclic AMP and cyclic GMP to construct a theory of growth control in normal epithelium and epithelium of the genetic disease psoriasis. Normal skin epithelium is avascular and in its constant exposure to the environment is subjected to rather "stringent step-down conditions" and as such is under cyclic AMP mediated negative pleiotypic control. Rapidly proliferating psoriasis epithelium is "relaxed" living "stepped-up conditions" and as such is under cyclic GMP mediated positive pleiotypic control.

INTRODUCTION

Although benign and malignant proliferative skin diseases afflict millions of people in this country, little is known about the molecular pathology of these disorders of growth control

and therapy is far from satisfactory. In general
the benign disorders of which psoriasis is prototypic are accompanied by accelerated proliferation of skin epithelium (1). The malignant disorders, primarily sun-induced basal and squamous
cell carcinomas, probably reproduce only somewhat
more rapidly than normal epithelium (1), but are
unable to stop dividing in response to physiological signals. The tremendous morbidity of these
diseases, the opportunity to compare benign and
malignant proliferation originating from the same
cell type, and the ready accessibility of tissue
biopsies from both mice and men prompted us to
investigate the molecular basis of common proliferative skin disease.

Our current research, begun in the fall of
1970, was initiated on the basis of earlier work
of others and the recent work of Ryan and Heidrick, a summary of which follows:

1) Bullough and Laurence at the University of
   London in 1961 showed that epinephrine inhibited (2):

   a) G_2 phase of the cell cycle in an in
      vitro assay
   b) epidermal cell division in an in vivo
      system

2) Epinephrine raised the cyclic AMP levels in
   many tissues (3)

3) Ryan and Heidrick in 1968 showed that cyclic
   AMP inhibited tumor cells in vitro (4); Burk
   had shown that polyoma viral transformed
   cells have reduced adenylate cyclase activity (5)

4) Glycogen accumulates in rapidly dividing
   skin epithelium (such as psoriasis) (6-9)

5) Epinephrine promotes glycogenolysis via cyclic AMP accumulation (3)

327

6) Iversen of Oslo had suggested a role for cyclic AMP in epithelial differentiation but
did not consider glycogen accumulation (10)

With these facts and speculations we constructed
the working hypothesis as shown in Fig. 1. The
proposition was that in normal epithelium cyclic
AMP maintained a normal cell cycle speed and normal glycogen concentration. If epinephrine inhibited cell division by increasing the levels of
cyclic AMP, then an event which produced a decrease in the cyclic AMP levels might induce the
rapid proliferation of the epithelium and glycogen accumulation. This would explain the apparent paradox of an accumulation of an energy
source (glycogen) at a time when large quantities
of energy are required for rapid proliferation.

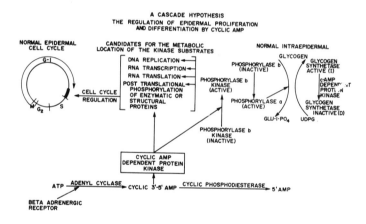

Figure 1. A depiction of the possible coordinate
control of two "superficially unrelated" metabolic sequences (the cell cycle and glycogen metabolism) by a
single "pleiotypic" molecular species—cyclic AMP.

Before examining the possibility of an actual or functional decrease in cyclic AMP levels in rapidly dividing epithelium using psoriasis as a prototype, it was necessary to prove that the hormone epinephrine (or isoproterenol (IPR) a more potent beta agonist analogue) could inhibit epithelial cell division via cyclic AMP elevation. Consequently, the format of this communication will be: 1) the fulfillment of the criteria of Robison, Butcher and Sutherland to prove that a particular hormonally mediated event, in this case, epithelial mitotic inhibition is mediated by cyclic AMP (11); 2) the presentation of data which strongly suggests that cyclic AMP is decreased in the lesions of psoriasis and data obtained in attempts to locate the cause for such a decrease; 3) our view of the role of cyclic nucleotides in epithelial cell proliferation.

EXPERIMENTAL

Cell cycle assay — The length of the entire cell cycle of the mouse ear epithelial cells is approximately 528 hours, S-phase approximately 30 hours and G_2 phase of 4.8 hours (12). A detailed description of the G_2 assay has been published (13), but the important features are that the drugs are added to a mouse ear fragment in vitro and mitotic figures in basal epithelial cells are enumerated after a four hour Colcemid collection period. Using this assay system the criteria of a cyclic AMP mediated event have been met. Experiments using a $G_1 \rightarrow S$ assay are in progress.

Epithelial procurement — The epithelium is obtained by a 30 second exposure to water at 55°C (13) or by a keratoming (14). Both techniques have been previously described in detail (13,14). With either method the purity of epithelium is monitored by paraffin or frozen section histology.

Cyclic AMP assays — We currently use the Gilman assay (15) although the assay of Brooker et al (16) was used in earlier experiments (17).

329

The TCA supernatant fractions containing the cyclic AMP are partially purified by anion exchange column chromatography. Cyclic AMP phosphodiesterase digestion results in the disappearance of 87% of what is assayed as cyclic AMP in the Brooker assay and 95% in the Gilman assay.

Adenylate cyclase assay — The details have been previously published (18). In our hands an ATP regenerating system is absolutely essential, the majority of ATP being hydrolyzed within five minutes without a regenerating system.

Phosphodiesterase assay — The phosphodiesterase activity in newborn rat epidermis and the high K_m enzyme in the psoriatic tissue were assayed using a modification of the radioisotope dilution method of Brooker et al (16). A two step incubation was used with the phosphodiesterase reaction being terminated by heating in a boiling water bath for one minute. After cooling to room temperature, the snake venom was added, incubated for ten minutes, and stopped with resin. The low K_m enzyme in psoriatic tissue was assayed according to the method of Beavo et al (19).

Radioautography — A slight modifiction of the methods of Baserga and Malamud were used (20).

Cyclic GMP analysis — This was performed in Professor Nelson Goldberg's laboratory by the fluorometric enzymic cycling technique which has been previously described (21).

Statistical design — See references 13 and 14 and caption of Table 1.

RESULTS AND DISCUSSION

Fulfillment of the four criteria of Robison, Butcher and Sutherland for cyclic AMP mediation of a hormone produced effect.

The first criterion is that the hormone in

question must increase the intracellular cyclic
AMP levels in intact cells, while inactive hormones should not increase cyclic AMP levels.
Using epithelial slices such as shown in Figure
2, the beta adrenergic agonist, isoproterenol
(IPR) at a concentration of 1×10^{-6}M produced a
205% increase in the cyclic AMP content of intact
cells (18). This rise was blocked by a ten-fold
excess of the beta adrenergic antagonist propranolol. All assays for cyclic AMP were conducted in the absence of any phosphodiesterase
inhibitors unless otherwise specified.

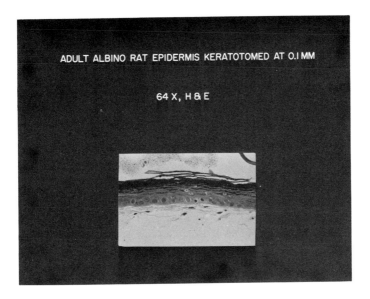

Figure 2. Mammalian epithelium (epidermis) of skin
with minimal mesenchymatous (dermal) contamination. This
tissue forms the barrier between the animal and the environment. This stratified squamous epithelium is composed
of four differentiating layers containing five cell types
(95% of the tissue volume is composed of keratinocytes,
the remaining four cell types being responsible for 5% of
the tissue). Such epithelium is avascular receiving nu-
trition by diffusion of nutrients from the dermis into the
epithelium.

Table 1 shows that IPR over a wide range of
concentrations inhibits cell division as measured
by the collection of cells undergoing mitosis during a five hour period. The cell cycle kinetics
are such that a five hour period of time is necessary for sufficient numbers of cells to move from
G_2 to the M phase of the cell cycle in control
tissue so that a statistically significant decrease in C-mitoses can be seen in experimental
tissue. The mechanism of G_2 delay (possible inhibition of mitotic spindle microtubular assembly
by cyclic AMP dependent protein kinase phosphorylation of tubulin subunits) which is seen as decreased C-mitoses at five hours, could occur five
minutes after addition of the IPR. This IPR induced inhibition of mitosis is blocked by propranolol (22).

INHIBITION OF EPIDERMAL MITOSIS BY A β-ADRENERGIC AGENT			
ADDITIONS TO EXPERIMENTAL FLASKS	MITOSES PER CM EPIDERMIS		MITOTIC INHIBITION (PERCENT)
	CONTROL	EXPERIMENTAL	
L-ISOPROTERENOL			
1×10^{-5} M	3.3 ± 0.2	1.4 ± 0.1	58*
1×10^{-6} M	3.5 ± 0.4	1.5 ± 0.2	57*
5×10^{-7} M	4.9 ± 1.6	3.1 ± 0.6	36*
1×10^{-7} M	2.6 ± 0.4	1.7 ± 0.2	36*
1×10^{-8} M	2.7 ± 0.5	2.1 ± 0.2	13

Table 1. Asterisks (*) indicate statistical significance at the .05 level or less using a Students t-
test in this and all other tables.

Vincent (23) had shown that the primarily
alpha agent norepinephrine did not inhibit epidermal mitosis. Somewhat erratic results have

been obtained with norepinephrine in our laboratory using the G_2 assay but significant inhibition occurs at $1 \times 10^{-5}M$ (higher or lower concentrations had no effect). In the sliced preparation, norepinephrine ($1 \times 10^{-5}M$) produced a 120% stimulation of cyclic AMP accumulation at three or six minutes. The increase in cyclic AMP was blocked by propranolol plus phentolamine but not by phentolamine alone. Phenylephrine had no effect on the levels of cyclic AMP. These data suggest that the epithelium has no alpha receptor but definitely contains a beta receptor (22).

The presence of a beta receptor has been independently confirmed by Brønstad et al (24). Whether the beta receptor is beta-1 or beta-2 is currently being investigated. The preceding data show that the isoproterenol induced accumulation of cyclic AMP does precede the event in question, namely, the inhibition of cell division. However, there is no unequivocal evidence to indicate that beta adrenergic stimulation participates in the physiological control of epidermal cell division. In our work we are using beta agonists as a tool to study the effects of elevated cyclic AMP levels on cell division. Epinephrine in concert with glucocorticoids may play some auxiliary role in controlling epithelial proliferation since there is a diurnal variation in epithelial DNA synthesis, mitosis (25) and cyclic AMP levels (26). It appears intuitively to us that nature must have produced a more effective way of regulating the fine control of epithelial proliferation than the circulating levels of adrenalin and glucocorticoids. Especially intriguing is the possibility that epithelial proliferation is under the neurobiological control of the intraepithelial argentaffin-like system, the Merkel cells (27). We will return to this matter of the physiological control of epithelial proliferation by hormones, nerves and other factors later.

The second criterion is that the hormone must stimulate adenylate cyclase in broken cell preparations of epithelium (11). It has been demonstrated that IPR (1 x 10^{-4}M) gives a statistically significant 40% stimulation of adenylate cyclase in the broken cell preparation (18). A 139% stimulation can be achieved with 0.016M NaF. The IPR stimulation is blocked with a ten-fold excess of propranolol. If one compares the results from the broken cell preparation and the slice preparation, a one hundred-fold excess of the IPR is needed to achieve approximately 20% of the stimulation obtained in the sliced tissue preparations. This illustrates dramatically that the epithelial beta receptors are exquisitely susceptible to homogenization and could explain the lack of catecholamine sensitivity of the adenylate cyclase in the results reported by Mier and Urselmann (28) using full thickness skin (an experimental approach with which we completely disagree due to the heterogeneity of skin). Marks and Rebien in Heidelberg (29) have confirmed our findings of a beta sensitive adenylate cyclase in broken cells prepared from skin epithelium. These investigators have tested a variety of hormones for their ability to stimulate broken cell epithelial cyclase. No stimulation was found with norepinephrine, glucagon, growth hormone, epidermal growth factor, serotonin, histamine, prostaglandin E_1 (PGE_1) and prostaglandin E_2 (PGE_2). These results must be interpreted cautiously due to the possibility of damage to the receptors. However, using epithelial slices with an intact beta receptor demonstrated for each experiment, our laboratory has found no cyclic AMP accumulation in the presence of phenylephrine, PGE_1, vasopressin, ACTH and glucagon (unpublished data). It seems quite possible that a beta receptor will be the only classic target tissue type receptor found on the epithelium of skin.

To meet the third criterion one must show that a classical phosphodiesterase (PDE) inhibitor is effective on the enzyme isolated from the tissue. Increased levels of cyclic AMP and occurrence of the metabolic effect should result

from incubation of the tissue with suboptimal concentrations of the hormone plus the inhibitor.
In Figure 3 it can be seen that theophylline will
inhibit the enzyme extracted from epithelium.
Theophylline by itself at several concentrations
will inhibit epidermal cell division (30). The
lowest effective dose of theophylline (5 x 10^{-4}M)
was combined with the three most dilute concentrations (see Table 1) of IPR. Table 2 shows that
the mitotic inhibition achieved at the two lowest
doses of IPR is significantly greater in the presence of theophylline indicating synergism. Marks
and Rebien have confirmed our findings that theophylline alone inhibits epidermal mitotic activity (31).

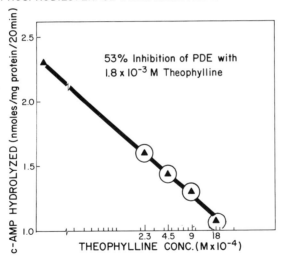

Figure 3. The phosphodiesterase activity in the
17,000xg supernatant was determined using a substrate concentration of 5 x 10^{-4}M cyclic AMP with increasing amounts
of theophylline.

SYNERGISTIC INHIBITION OF EPIDERMAL MITOSIS BY ISOPROTERENOL AND THEOPHYLLINE		
L-ISOPROTERENOL IN EXPT'L FLASKS	MITOSES PER CM EPIDERMIS CONTROL · · EXPERIMENTAL	MITOTIC INHIBITION % DECREASE
5×10^{-7} M	3.7 ± 0.4 · · 2.2 ± 0.1	41^*
1×10^{-7} M	4.1 ± 0.3 · · 2.3 ± 0.1	43^*
1×10^{-8} M	3.7 ± 0.4 · · 2.3 ± 0.1	38^*

5×10^{-4} M THEOPHYLLINE IN EXPL'T FLASKS; 19% INHIBITION.

Table 2

Lastly as a fourth criterion one should be able to mimic the physiological effect of the hormone by adding cyclic AMP to the cells exogenously. The effects of dibutyryl cyclic AMP (5×10^{-3}M to 5×10^{-7}M) on the inhibition of epidermal mitosis has been published (32). A dose response curve was obtained with a maximum of 76% to a 46% statistically significant response at 5×10^{-5}M. Inhibition was obtained with the two most dilute concentrations but the results were not statistically significant. Sodium butyrate or 5'AMP at millimolar concentrations had no effect on epidermal mitoses. Marks and Rebien have also confirmed the fact that dibutyryl cyclic AMP inhibits epidermal mitosis in a G_2 assay over a concentration range similar to ours (31).

These data from our laboratory lead us to three conclusions: 1) the IPR and epinephrine inhibition or delay of the G_2 phase of the skin epithelial cell cycle may be mediated by cyclic AMP; 2) this epithelium probably does not have an

336

alpha receptor; and 3) an increase in epithelial cyclic AMP concentration above some "critical" threshold will probably produce a block in cell division. This has important therapeutic implications to be mentioned later.

A corollary of the above statements would be: a compound which lowers cyclic AMP levels might result in an increase in the rate of epithelial cell division. In our early deliberations it was considered that histamine might be a candidate for such a role since imidazole compounds are known to stimulate cyclic AMP phosphodiesterase (33) and histamine has also been associated with rapidly dividing tissues (34).

However, only very high concentrations of histamine ($5 \times 10^{-2}M$) were found to produce any significant stimulation of cyclic AMP phosphodiesterase activity when measured in a crude epithelial extract at pH 7.5 (35). At this same concentration a stimulation of mitosis with cell damage did occur. A dose response curve with histamine concentrations from $5 \times 10^{-2}M$ to $1 \times 10^{-4}M$ was constructed using the G_2 assay. A 837% increase in mitotic activity occurred when $3.5 \times 10^{-2}M$ histamine was incubated with the epithelial tissue with no apparent cell damage (35). Whether such concentrations are achieved in pathological tissue is unknown and the possibility that it may have effects under physiological conditions beyond its cell membrane receptor(s) directly on particulate or cytoplasmic cyclic AMP phosphodiesterase activity remains to be established. Rather than suggest that histamine is involved in any physiological or pathological epithelial situations, we are content to consider histamine as a tool and would like to suggest that it may lower cyclic AMP levels in epithelium and thus stimulate mitotic activity.

An alternative explanation of the histamine effect involves cyclic GMP. Although histamine can stimulate cyclic AMP accumulation in some tissues (36), in others it has been found to increase both cyclic AMP and cyclic GMP levels (37) or those of cyclic GMP alone (see footnote 1). Furthermore, an increased level of cyclic GMP is associated with mitogen induced lymphocyte proliferation (38). However there is also ample evidence that in abnormal circumstances such as tumor cells in vitro (39-44) that the rate of cell division and cyclic AMP levels are in general inversely proportional. Whether normal epithelium must lower its cyclic AMP below some "permissive" level in order to repair a simple wound remains a problem for the future.

Cyclic AMP and Cyclic GMP in Psoriasis

General — The apparently paradoxical relationship between rapid epithelial proliferation and glycogen accumulation is not unique to psoriasis. If this paradox can be explained by decreased cyclic AMP levels, then one might expect to find depressed cyclic AMP levels in other proliferative disorders of skin epithelium. Figure 4-A shows the markedly increased labelling index in epithelium of psoriasis in comparison with uninvolved areas (Figure 4-B). The increased glycogen content can be seen in Figure 4-C in comparison with uninvolved areas (Figure 4-D). Biochemically the glycogen content of involved areas is five-fold that of uninvolved areas (7). Autoradiographically there is a twelve-fold acceleration in the rate of the cell cycle in comparison with normal epithelium (1).

Figure 5 shows the thickened proliferative epithelium of involved atopic dermatitis which clearly shows a marked accumulation of glycogen

---

Footnote 1 — Personal communication from Dr. Guenter Schultz and Dr. Joel Hardman who have found histamine induced contraction of intestinal smooth muscle to be associated with increases in tissue cyclic GMP and not in cyclic AMP levels.

although the increase has not been measured biochemically. Psoriasis can be used as a model of
abnormal epithelial proliferation since a variety
of skin disorders (psoriasis, atopic dermatitis,
wounded skin epithelium, ultraviolet light exposed skin, and squamous cell cancers) as well as
superficially damaged corneal, esophageal, and
gall bladder epithelia have increased glycogen and
cell cycle rates (45). In these disorders the kinetics of glycogen accumulation occurring within a
few hours of damage and the initiation of DNA synthesis followed by mitosis occurring many hours
later argues for a release of cells from G_1 or G_0
to repair damage following injury. If the damage
released only a G_2 population there would be no
increase in DNA synthesis and the mitotic wave
would occur within four or five hours.

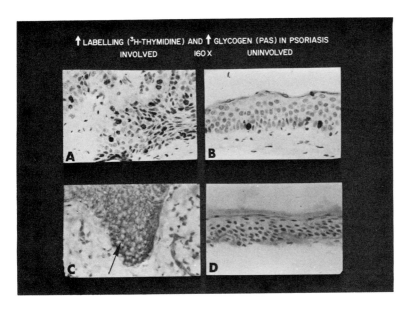

Figure 4. The increased labelling index of psoriasis
epithelium (A) can be compared with uninvolved epithelium
(B). The arrow in panel C points to darkly staining amylase susceptible material which is glycogen. Virtually no
such material is seen in uninvolved tissue (D).

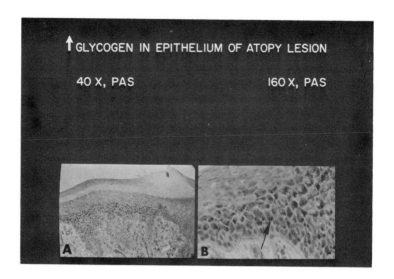

Figure 5. Low (A) and high (B) power views of frozen sections of atopic epithelium. The marked accumulation
of darkly staining amylase susceptible materical can be seen
at both low and high (tip of arrow) power.

An effect of cyclic AMP on the G_1 phase of
the cell cycle is being investigated at the present time by using the co-carcinogen, tetradeca-
nolyl phorbol acetate (TPA) which is known to
stimulate the cells from G_1 to the S phase of the
cell cycle. Intraperitoneal injections of IPR
have been given to mice painted with TPA in an
effort to block the flow of cells from $G_1 \to S$. Although marked rises in intraepithelial cyclic AMP
were measured as a result of the IPR injections,
the $G_1 \to S$ delay has not been consistently demonstrated in our laboratory (data not shown).
These studies are being continued with special
considerations being given to diurnal variations
in intraepithelial cyclic AMP levels which may
affect the system.

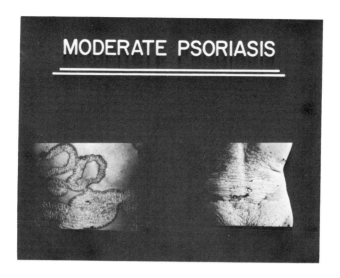

Figure 6

Psoriasis — A patient having psoriasis of moderate severity is shown in Figure 6. The global prevalence ranges from 1 to 3% of the population without any predilection for either sex (46) and may appear at any age. The features of psoriasis which are especially pertinent to our approach to this disease are summarized in Figure 7. The clinical essence of psoriasis is epithelial hyperplasia although the primary molecular location of the cause may not be epithelial (47). The aim of our research is to understand the mechanism of this hyperplasia rather than the cause due to the controversy over the exact genetic nature of the disease.

Although altered differentiation is a prominent feature of the involved epithelium, our view is that this is secondary to the rapid cell division, but the possibility exists that a block in epithelial specialization which gives rise to the aberrant morphology of psoriatic epithelium could result in compensatory cellular hyperplasia. These considerations plus the localized nature of this disease suggest that the rapid proliferation is the result of perturbations in those molecular mechanisms which exert fine control over the cell cycle.

FEATURES OF PSORIASIS PERTINENT TO ITS MOLECULAR BASIS

Epithelial Hyperplasia

Altered Differentiation

Genetic Disease

Lesions are Sporadic and Self Limiting

Lesions can be Produced by Damage to Skin

Glycogen Accumulation in Epithelium

Figure 7

Psoriasis and cyclic AMP — Figure 8 illustrates our model for the molecular basis of the rapid epithelial cell cycle kinetics of psoriasis which may also pertain to those rapidly dividing glycogen containing epithelial disorders previously mentioned. In summary an actual or functional decrease in cyclic AMP in the lesion could account for the twelve-fold accelerated cell cycle and the five-fold increase in glycogen via a suboptimal cyclic AMP dependent protein kinase activation.

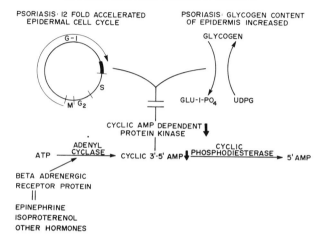

POSSIBLE MOLECULAR BASIS OF THE RAPID
EPIDERMAL CELL CYCLE KINETICS OF PSORIASIS

Figure 8

To test this hypothesis involved and uninvolved epithelium was removed from psoriasis patients and volunteers without a history of psoriasis as previously described (14). Figure 9-A
shows an ideal cleavage with 5 to 10% dermal contamination. Figure 9-B shows a specimen with more
dermis than epithelium due to inadvertent excessive pressure by the operator. Both the normal
and uninvolved psoriatic epithelium are similar
histologically and have similar procurement problems. The psoriasis lesions present a different
problem since the plaques vary in depth. Figure
10-A is an ideal biopsy whereas Figure 10-B and C
are unacceptable. In Figure 10-B much of the proliferative compartment remains on the patient
leaving a larger proportion of dead scale for one
to analyze chemically while Figure 10-C has as

much mesenchyme (dermis) as epithelium.

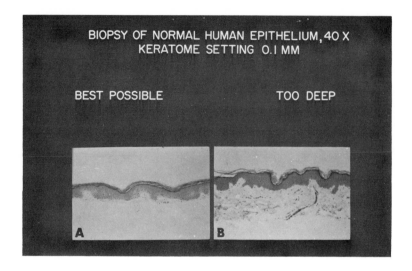

Figure 9

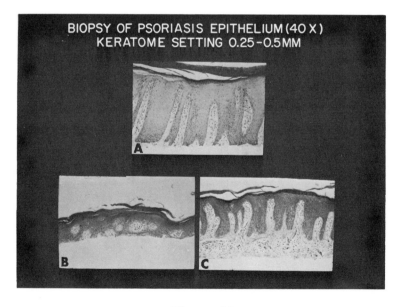

Figure 10

All specimens are examined histologically and must resemble Figures 9-A and 10-A to be acceptable for biochemical analysis. Even with these precautions it is very difficult to make meaningful biochemical comparisons between involved epithelium (Figure 10-A) and uninvolved epithelium (Figure 9-A) with correct depths of the biopsies. This has been discussed in detail in a previous report (14) and will be only summarized here:

1) A comparison between normal and pathological tissue (almost equivalent to two different types of tissues);
2) Increased and variable amount of scale on the lesion;
3) Increased yield of assayable protein from the lesion (22% increase per mg wet weight);
4) Increased yield of DNA from the lesion (9% increase per mg wet weight);
5) Increased dermal contamination via the unavoidable dermal papillae in the lesions.

Since a satisfactory data base is difficult to obtain we have used three—wet weight, protein and DNA. For simplicity and because the DNA values show the least variation between involved and uninvolved areas, the results will be expressed in terms of DNA values for this communication.

Decreased cyclic AMP in psoriasis — The biochemical data given in Table 3 were obtained from specimens which were histologically acceptable according to the above criteria, with an average keratome depth of 0.350 mm. The decrease in cyclic AMP in involved epithelium (IE) versus uninvolved epithelium (UE) of psoriasis patients is highly significant (p=0.001, 36% decrease) using a paired data design. It is of interest that the UE has significantly higher cyclic AMP levels than normal epithelium of controls. The reason for this is not apparent at the present time, but is under current investigation. The data derived by two different cyclic AMP assays in a total of 50 patients thus support the hypothesis put forward in Figure 8.

cAMP LEVELS IN SNAP FROZEN EPITHELIUM OF 50 PSORIATIC AND 32 CONTROL SUBJECTS				
Method of Assay	pmoles of c-AMP/μg DNA PSORIATIC PATIENTS		% DECREASE	pmoles of cAMP/μg DNA CONTROL PATIENTS
	Uninvolved	Involved		
BROOKER (N=25)	0.7±0.1	0.4±0.1	43*	0.5±0.1(N=25)
GILMAN (N=25)	1.1±0.1	0.7±0.1	36*	0.6±0.1(N=7)

Table 3

Figure 11 lists the possible explanations which have occurred to us to explain this decrease. We have previously discussed item 4 and believe that the use of three data bases (wet weight, DNA and protein) makes it unlikely that the data are a function of an unstable denominator. In order to minimize item 5, we have used the following technical quality controls when assaying cyclic AMP in histologically acceptable specimens: The cyclic AMP determination for each sample was conducted in duplicate at three different dilutions. The protein or DNA determinations are also performed at three different dilutions of the homogenate. All calculations are performed on the IBM 360/67 computer and the three (DNA and protein) and six determinations (cyclic AMP) of a given sample of both involved and uninvolved epithelium must all agree within 5 to 10% in each patient to be acceptable for biological consideration. The cyclic AMP is partially purified by anion exchange column chroma-

tography prior to assay and an overall recovery
of at least 50% is necessary. After cyclic phosphodiesterase digestion, at least 87 to 95% of
the assayable cyclic AMP was hydrolyzed.

POSSIBLE EXPLANATIONS FOR " DECREASED CYCLIC AMP" IN PSORIASIS

1. A GENETIC OR TEMPORARY DECREASE (↓)
   IN ADENYL CYCLASE ACTIVITY

2. A GENETIC OR TEMPORARY INCREASE (↑)
   IN PDE ACTIVITY

3. CYCLIC AMP DIFFUSION OUT OF EPIDERMIS

4. FAULTY DATA BASE (MISLEADING DENOMINATOR)

5. COMPLETE TECHNICAL INCOMPETENCE

6. AN INCREASE IN CYCLIC GMP IN PSORIATIC
   LESIONS

Figure 11

Item 1 of Figure 11 is difficult to approach
experimentally and at the same time obtain meaningful results. A decrease in the specific activity of isolated adenylate cyclase could be interpreted as a true decrease in activity, a pref-
erential loss of activity due to increased membrane fragility to homogenization in the involved
tissue or to an increase in enzymatically inactive
protein due to the increased quantity of dead and
dying scale.

Furthermore, the use of radioactive adenine
and the prelabelling technique (48) in adenylate
cyclase assays also contains variables that are
difficult to measure. The uninvolved and involved

psoriasis appear almost as two different types of tissue. One must assume that the adenine penetrates to the same degree that it is incorporated into the ATP pool and that the specific activities of the ATP pool that serves as substrate for the adenylate cyclase are the same in both the IE and UE. Since it seemed quite unlikely that these conditions would exist another approach was taken.

Figure 11, items 1 and 2 have been examined in slice preparations of normal epithelium in comparison with IE and UE of psoriasis patients. This design maintains an intact beta receptor, a possibility for prostaglandin modulation, as well as an intact adenylate cyclase and cyclic phosphodiesterase (cyclic AMP—PDE). The epithelium was removed from the patient or control volunteer, placed in saline on ice until reaching the laboratory. The total length of time between the clinic and completion of the slicing in the laboratory consumed approximately 45 minutes. After a ten minute preincubation at 30°C, 1×10^{-6}M IPR was added to a portion of the tissue. After 3 minutes of additional incubation the samples with and without IPR treatment were frozen in liquid nitrogen. The cyclic AMP content of each of the samples was then determined. If less cyclic AMP was found in IE versus UE, then the defect would lie in the receptor-adenylate cyclase complex, an overly active cyclic AMP—PDE since no phosphodiesterase inhibitors were used or as Figure 11—item 3 suggests, diffusion from IE into the medium in excess of that occurring in UE.

A highly significant 128% stimulation by IPR in control subjects was obtained with the slice preparation as shown in Table 4.

Using the same type of experimental design with the psoriasis tissue, the uninvolved epithelium gave very similar results but the involved epithelium had a much lower percent stimulation as shown in Table 5.

348

cAMP LEVELS IN THE EPITHELIUM OF 16 NORMAL SUBJECTS BEFORE AND AFTER BETA-ADRENERGIC STIMULATION

picomoles of cAMP/μg DNA		% STIMULATION
without Isoproterenol	with Isoproterenol	
0.9 ± 0.2	2.1 ± 0.4	128*

Table 4

cAMP IN THE EPITHELIUM OF 23 PSORIATIC PATIENTS BEFORE AND AFTER BETA-ADRENERGIC STIMULATION

PSORIATIC EPITHELIUM	pmoles of cAMP/μg DNA		% STIMULATION
	without Isoproterenol	with Isoproterenol	
Uninvolved	0.6 ± 0.1	1.3 ± 0.2	117*
Involved	1.1 ± 0.2	1.5 ± 0.2	36*

Table 5

If one examines these data more closely, particularly the IE cyclic AMP levels without IPR in comparison with the UE cyclic AMP levels, then it becomes apparent that the baseline cyclic AMP level
probably rose in the IE and not in the UE between
the time the biopsy was taken and the incubation
terminated in liquid nitrogen.

Further examination of the data in Table 5
shows that the concentration of cyclic AMP in the
involved sample with IPR is slightly higher than
the amount present in the corresponding sample of
uninvolved tissue. Therefore it seems to us unlikely that the beta receptor or adenylate cyclase
is defective genetically or that cyclic AMP—PDE is
genetically overactive, because either situation
would lead to a less total accumulation of cyclic
AMP in IE versus UE. The presence of an inhibitor
of adenylate cyclase or activator of cyclic AMP—
PDE may occur temporarily in the lesion in vivo
but is less active in vitro. However, one must
still consider the possibility that the 25% dermal
contamination in these lesions is modifying the
values. In contrast to these results, Hsia et al
(49) reported a 50%↓ in the specific activity of
the adenylate cyclase obtained from the involved
area of a psoriatic patient versus the uninvolved
area. The same type of results were reported
using the prelabelling technique (^{3}H-adenine incorporation into ATP) for 11 involved and 3 uninvolved areas (49). For the reasons cited earlier,
these results are also open to other interpretations. These issues could perhaps be resolved by
immunocytochemistry as recently described by Siggins et al (50).

Cyclic AMP phosphodiesterase — Since an apparent gross defect in the beta receptor—adenylate
cyclase activity could not be demonstrated, the
cyclic AMP—PDE activity was examined in IE versus
UE. Preliminary results indicate the presence of
two enzymes with K_m's of approximately 5×10^{-5}M
and 1×10^{-6}M. The maximum catalytic capacity of
the soluble enzyme at a concentration of 5×10^{-4}M

cyclic AMP was approximately the same in IE versus UE as seen in Table 6. The cyclic AMP—PDE specific activity in a homogenate with several concentrations of cyclic AMP as substrate showed no difference in five patients between IE and UE. Thus the preliminary work suggests that there is no alteration in the V_{max} of the 17,000xg supernatant high K_m enzyme and no apparent alteration in the K_m or the V_{max} of the low K_m enzyme as assayed in a homogenate. Although a more rigorous examination of both adenylate cyclase and cyclic AMP—PDE is now in progress with both normal controls and psoriatic patients, it seems unlikely that a major defect will be detected in vitro. The possibility does exist that the psoriasis patient did inherit an altered adenylate cyclase (characterized by a higher K_m for ATP) or cyclic AMP—PDE (characterized by a lower K_m for cAMP) or an altered allosteric binding site on either enzyme which can be detected by a comparison with normal volunteers. Inherited defects resulting in abnormal allosteric regulation could result in altered enzymatic activity in vivo which would not be detected in vitro unless one includes the appropriate allosteric inhibitor or activator in the reaction mixture.

SOLUBLE CYCLIC PHOSPHODIESTERASE ACTIVITY IN
EIGHTEEN PSORIATIC EPITHELIA WITH
5×10^{-4} M c-AMP AS SUBSTRATE

pmoles of c-AMP Hydrolyzed/10 mins.	PSORIATIC EPITHELIA		DECREASED ACTIVITY
	Uninvolved	Involved	
per μg DNA	171±33	141±77	17%

Table 6

At present there is no experimental evidence
in our laboratory to explain the decrease in cyclic AMP in the snap frozen lesions. Some attempts have been made to determine the flow of cyclic AMP out of the cells. Although our data make
this seem unlikely, an increased exit of cyclic
AMP in IE versus UE is still a possibility since
our assays for cyclic AMP in the medium give in-
consistent results and therefore do not meet our
criteria for quality control as described earlier.

In the spring of 1972 we met Professor Nelson Goldberg who told us of the evidence he was
accumulating in support of the concept that cyclic GMP may be involved in promoting cellular
events that are antagonistic to those promoted
when tissue levels of cyclic AMP are elevated.
Particularly relevant were the results of some
cell transformation experiments he had conducted
in collaboration with Dr. John Hadden at the University of Minnesota. Hadden and Goldberg had
found striking increases in the levels of cellular
cyclic GMP concentrations associated with PHA and
Concanavalin A induced lymphocyte transformation
(38). This observation was, in a sense, consistent with the findings of Whitfield et al (51)
that cyclic GMP in very low concentrations could
directly stimulate thymic lymphoblast proliferation. However, there is a fundamental difference
in the findings of Whitfield et al (51) and Hadden et al (38) because the latter investigators
found no concomitant increase in cyclic AMP levels
in the first thirty minutes after exposure to purified mitogens, whereas Whitfield et al (51) concluded that the cyclic GMP induced proliferation
they observed was apparently due to a cyclic GMP
induced elevation of cellular cyclic AMP levels.
This would be clearly different than the situation in psoriasis also because if the levels
of cyclic GMP were to be elevated in this condition, the change in cyclic AMP concentration is
an unequivocal decrease. Because of the findings
of Hadden et al (38) we wondered whether a chronically dividing psoriasis epithelium might be anal-

ogous to mitogen induced lymphocyte proliferation. Furthermore, even though a decreased cyclic AMP level did not occur in the lymphocyte, a rise in cyclic GMP might decrease cyclic AMP in another system in vivo which has been shown may be the case in heart muscle (52). This could be brought about theoretically either via the stimulation by cyclic GMP of cyclic AMP—PDE which Beavo, Hardman and Sutherland (19) had previously shown in vitro or as suggested by Goldberg et al (53), by a decrease in the GTP concentration in a compartment of the membrane. Rodbell and his colleagues (54) have shown a GTP requirement for optimal hormone activation of adenylate cyclase activity in isolated membrane preparations.

We provided samples of IE and UE, which had been monitored as previously discussed, to Professor Goldberg and Mari Haddox who analyzed the samples for cyclic GMP and obtained the data shown in Table 7. The 94% increase in cyclic GMP levels in IE versus UE is highly significant statistically (p=.001). Whether this increase is derived from the rapidly dividing epithelial cells and not the 25% contaminating dermal papillae is unknown. The fibroblasts in this contaminating tissue do not divide rapidly and hence we suspect that the elevated cyclic GMP level is most probably epithelial in origin. The role of cyclic GMP in epithelial proliferation and its ability to stimulate the epithelial cyclic AMP—PDE as well as the effect of GTP on epithelial adenylate cyclase activity are under current investigation.

c-GMP LEVELS IN THE SNAP FROZEN EPITHELIUM OF 12 PSORIATIC PATIENTS		
femtomoles / µg DNA		%
Uninvolved	Involved	Increase
6.1 ± 1.0	11.8 ± 3.4	94*

Table 7

Cyclic Nucleotides in Epithelial Proliferation

Goldberg and his colleagues have proposed a "dualism" theory of biological control through opposing actions of cyclic GMP and cyclic AMP (53, 55). In this framework those situations associated with a fall in cyclic AMP level would be associated with an opposing rise in cyclic GMP. In the case of cell proliferation, Hadden et al (38) proposed that the rise in cyclic GMP may be the primary and active signal, while the fall in cyclic AMP, if it should occur, would be permissive. Although in the case of psoriasis it is not known whether cyclic GMP rises before cyclic AMP falls, we wish to interpret our data in terms of Goldberg's "dualism" concept as it applies to a bidirectionally regulated system (56).

For normal epithelial homeostasis to prevail the effects of cyclic GMP and cyclic AMP must be balanced. Our concept of the role of cyclic GMP and cyclic AMP in the fine control of epithelial proliferation and differentiation is shown in

Figure 12. If an imbalance occurs in favor of
cyclic GMP, cell proliferation may occur in which
case the degree of tissue specialization would be
quantitatively reduced. It is possible that if
cyclic AMP is not depressed below some critical
level, the proliferative stimulus that may be provided by cyclic GMP would not become manifest.
In this context, in epithelium cyclic GMP may be
the active proliferative trigger whereas cyclic
AMP plays a permissive role. A corollary of this
is that if one maintains cyclic AMP above a threshold level, cell proliferation will not proceed.
If the ratio of cyclic AMP to cyclic GMP is high,
one would expect maximum induction of cell specialization and a quantitative reduction of cell
proliferation.

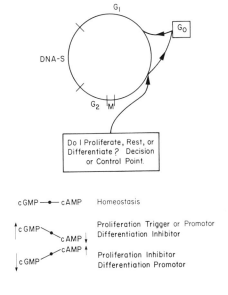

BALANCE BETWEEN EPITHELIAL PROLIFERATION AND DIFFERENTIATION
REGULATED BY cAMP AND cGMP-A HYPOTHESIS

Figure 12

355

In psoriasis cyclic GMP is maintained at a relatively high level and cyclic AMP at a low level. We are proposing that the rapid epithelial proliferation in this disorder is intimately associated with an imbalanced cyclic GMP—cyclic AMP ratio to the extent that in the absence of this disturbance the rapid proliferation would not be possible.

If such an imbalance serves as a basis for rapid epithelial proliferation, three possible chemical mediators are: 1)cholinergic transmitters; 2) prostaglandins; and 3) histamine. It was first shown by George et al (52) that cholinergic stimulation promotes cellular cyclic GMP accumulation. In 1955 Szodoray and Einleitung (57) claim to have found an excess of acetylcholine and increased acetylcholinesterase in psoriasis lesions in comparison with normal. One might suggest a cholinergic-adrenergic imbalance in the lesion of psoriasis to account for our data. Although we are aware of no measurements of sympathetic mediators in the skin of psoriasis, the claimed excess of acetylcholine could explain the elevated cyclic GMP levels. In essence we are postulating a proliferative role for cholinergic (cyclic GMP) stimuli and an inhibitory role for adrenergic (cyclic AMP) stimuli. Although such a proposal may seem to be highly speculative it should be noted that Needham arrived at essentially the same postulate from published data in his classic treatise on regeneration and wound healing in 1952 (58) years before the discovery of cyclic AMP and cyclic GMP.

Altered prostaglandin biosynthesis could account for the imbalance in the ratio of cyclic nucleotides. As shown in Figure 13, prostaglandin E_2 (PGE_2) will cause an increase in cyclic AMP levels in skin epithelium. The modulation of cyclic AMP biosynthesis might be a physiological role of PGE_2 in epithelium since there appears to be epithelial hyperplasia in the skin of the essential fatty acid deficient rat which can be normalized by the topical application of PGE$_2$ (59). Perhaps it does so by raising intraepithelial cyclic AMP levels. This animal model and the demonstrated rise in cyclic GMP in uterine (53) and venous (56) tissue in response to prostaglandin F$_{2\alpha}$ suggests that a shift in prostaglandin biosynthesis in favor of PGF$_{2\alpha}$ and away from PGE$_2$ could tip the cyclic GMP—cyclic AMP ratio in favor of cyclic GMP with attendant proliferation.

Lastly, elevated levels of histamine are associated with rapidly dividing tissues (34), histamine will cause hair epithelium to grow in vitro (60), can stimulate epithelial mitosis (35), and can stimulate cyclic GMP accumulation without elevating those of cyclic AMP (see footnote 1 earlier in paper). We are aware of no reported measurements of histamine in epithelium of psoriasis.

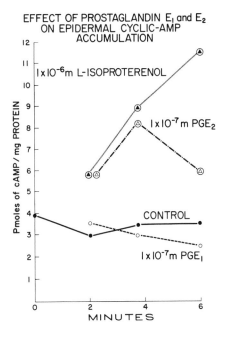

EFFECT OF PROSTAGLANDIN E$_1$ and E$_2$
ON EPIDERMAL CYCLIC-AMP
ACCUMULATION

Figure 13

The decreased level of cyclic AMP in rapidly
dividing epithelium of psoriasis seems analogous
to the low cyclic AMP levels which Pastan and his
coworkers (39,41) and Sheppard (40) have demonstrated in rapidly dividing "malignant" cells in
vitro. Whether this apparent analogy has biological significance is a problem for the future as
we have not examined endogenous cyclic AMP levels
in malignant epithelium and psoriasis does not undergo spontaneous malignant transformation. However it is interesting that an apparently benign
phenotype can be conferred on transformed cells
in culture by treating them with cyclic AMP (61,
62). Other phenotypic changes can be conferred
on benign cells (63,64). In very preliminary
single blind studies we have applied the cyclic
AMP elevating agent, papaverine, to epithelium of
psoriasis with restoration of a clinically normal
epithelial phenotype (unpublished data). When cyclic AMP is removed from the culture medium of
transformed cells, the "malignant" phenotype reappears (62,65). When we stop the application of
papaverine, the lesions reappear in the same area
or elsewhere days to weeks later. We propse that
this reappearance occurs in response to whatever
stimulus causes the cyclic AMP level to fall.

If our preliminary observations with papaverine can be substantiated by appropriate double
blind studies which are currently in progress, it
would be of interest to know the mechanism of cyclic AMP action in psoriasis. Does cyclic AMP
limit proliferation, induce differentiation or
both. The extensive experimental demonstrations
of Prasad and coworkers (66-70), of Prasad and
Sheppard (71), of Furmanski et al (72) and of
Johnson and Pastan (73,74) show that both can occur.

As mentioned previously, the disease appears
and disappears and then reappears spontaneously.
Therefore, although the genetic defect which
causes the disease is permanent, the defect responsible for the clinical proliferative lesion

of psoriasis must be reversible. A decrease in cyclic AMP could be the result of a temporary (quantitative) reduction in the biosynthesis of cell surface or cell—cell recognition sites (the differentiation antigens of Scheid et al (75)) which might be modulators of the intracellular concentration of cyclic AMP. Alternatively, a quantitative and transient change in the cell surface or membrane could facilitate the entry of nutrients into cells as suggested by Sheppard (76) and Holley (77). Facilitated nutrient transport could control cyclic AMP levels via allosteric regulation without necessarily altering the biosynthesis of adenylate cyclase or cyclic AMP phosphodiesterase.

Many of the foregoing speculations regarding the role of cyclic nucleotides in growth control would also seem to fit the model of negative and positive pleiotypism proposed by Hershko et al (78), Mamont et al (79) and by Tomkins and Gelehrter (80). These investigators proposed that cyclic AMP serves as a pleiotypic mediator. Our hypothesis which is modeled after that of Hadden et al (38) would extend the proposal of Tomkins in that cyclic AMP would be the negative pleiotypic mediator and cyclic GMP the positive pleiotypic mediator in our system—psoriasis. In normal human epithelium cyclic AMP dominates keeping the epithelium under "step—down" conditions. In psoriasis positive pleiotypism is in effect, the epithelium operating under "stepped—up" conditions, possibly mediated by cyclic GMP. Whether one must also have a concomitant reduction in cyclic AMP levels in positive pleiotypism is a pertinent consideration also.

The preceding discussion is obviously a grossly over—simplified concept of probably the most complicated problem of modern cell and molecular biology—the understanding of growth control. However, it would appear that if we knew why the rapidly dividing cells of psoriasis have temporarily reduced levels of cyclic AMP, whereas cancer may have permanently reduced levels, we would be closer to an understanding of both disorders. This idea is not new, similar thoughts regarding psoriasis and growth control having been reviewed by Robison (81) and by Professor Potter (82) in his treatise on abnormal growth—the challenge of diversity.

This investigation was supported in part by the National Institute of Arthritis and Metabolic Diseases research grant AM 15740-01, the Irene Heinz and John LaPorte Given Foundation, General Research Support grant RR-05383-09, Babcock Dermatological Endowment Fund and American Cancer Society institutional research grant IN-40J and grants NB-05979 and HE-07939. We wish to thank Mrs. Branca Baic, David Chernin, Miss Kathleen Engelhard and Emmet Hayes for expert technical assistance. We are especially indebted to Dr. Nancy Colburn for her suggestions in the preparation of this manuscript.

REFERENCES

(1)   G. D. Weinstein and J. L. McCullough, in: Annual Review of Medicine (Annual Reviews, Inc., Palo Alto, Calif., 1973) in press.

(2)   W. S. Bullough and E. B. Laurence, Proc. Royal Society of London, B. 154 (1961) 540.

(3)   G. A. Robison, R. W. Butcher and E. W. Sutherland, in: Annual Review of Biochemistry, ed. P. D. Boyer (Annual Reivews, Inc., Palo Alto, Calif., 1968) p 149.

(4)   W. L. Ryan and M. L. Heidrick, Science 162 (1968) 1484.

(5)   R. R. Bürk, Nature (London) 219 (1968) 1272.

(6)   O. Braun-Falco, Ann. N.Y. Acad. Sci. 73 (1958) 936.

(7)   K. M. Halprin, A. Ohkawara and V. Levine, Arch. Dermatol. (1973) in press.

(8)   W. C. Lobitz, Jr., D. Brophy, A. E. Larner and F. Daniels, Jr., Arch. Dermatol. 86 (1962) 207.

(9)   R. W. Goltz, R. M. Fusaro and J. Jarvis, J. Invest. Dermatol. 31 (1958) 331.

(10)   O. H. Iversen, in: Homeostatic Regulators, ed. G. E. W. Wolstenholme and J. Knight (J. & A. Churchill Ltd. 1969) p 29.

(11)   G. A. Robison, R. W. Butcher and E. W. Sutherland, in: Cyclic AMP (Academic Press, N.Y. 1971) p 36.

(12)   A.W. Pollister, in: Physical Techniques in Biological Research, second edition (Academic Press, N.Y. 1969) p 123.

(13) J. M. Marrs and J. J. Voorhees, J. Invest. Dermatol. 56 (1971) 174.

(14) J. J. Voorhees, E. A. Duell, L. J. Bass, J. A. Powell and E. R. Harrell, Arch. Dermatol. 105 (1972) 695.

(15) A. G. Gilman, Proc. Nat. Acad. Sci. U.S. 67 (1970) 305.

(16) G. Brooker, L. J. Thomas, Jr. and M. M. Appleman. Biochemistry 7 (1968) 4177.

(17) J. A. Powell, E. A. Duell and J. J. Voorhees, Arch. Dermatol. 104 (1971) 359.

(18) E. A. Duell, J. J. Voorhees, W. H. Kelsey and E. Hayes, Arch. Dermatol. 104 (1971) 601.

(19) J. A. Beavo, J. G. Hardman and E. W. Sutherland, J. Biol. Chem. 246 (1971) 3841.

(20) R. Baserga and D. Malamud, in: Modern Methods in Experimental Pathology. Autoradiography: Techniques and Application (Harper and Row, N.Y. 1969) p 17.

(21) N. D. Goldberg and A. G. O'Toole, in: Methods of Biochemical Analysis, Vol. 20, ed. D. Glick (John Wiley & Sons, Inc. N.Y. 1971) p 1.

(22) E. A. Duell, W. H. Kelsey, E. Hayes and J. J. Voorhees, in preparation.

(23) N. H. Vincent, Fed. Proc. 29 (1970) 742.

(24) G. O. Brønstad, K. Elgjo and I. Øye, Nature (New Biol.) 233 (1971) 78.

(25) D. D. Grube, H. Auerbach and A. M. Brues, Cell Tissue Kinet. 3 (1970) 363.

(26) F. Marks and W. Grimm, Nature (New Biol.) 240 (1972) 178.

(27) P. H. J. Nafstad, Z. Zellforsch. 122 (1971) 528.

(28) P. D. Mier and E. Urselmann, Brit. J. Dermatol. 83 (1970) 359.

(29) F. Marks and W. Rebien, Biochim. Biophys. Acta 284 (1972) 556.

(30) E. A. Duell, L. J. Bass, W. H. Kelsey and J. J. Voorhees, in preparation.

(31) F. Marks and W. Rebien, Naturwissenschaften 59 (1972) 41.

(32) J. J. Voorhees, E. A. Duell and W. H. Kelsey, Arch. Dermatol. 105 (1972) 384.

(33) R. W. Butcher and E. W. Sutherland, J. Biol. Chem. 237 (1962) 1244.

(34) G. Kahlson and E. Rosengren, in: Biogenesis and Physiology of Histamine (Williams and Wilkins Co., Baltimore, 1971) p 235.

(35) J. J. Voorhees, E. A. Duell, L. J. Bass, J. A. Powell and E. R. Harrell, J. Invest. Dermatol. 59 (1972) 114.

(36) G. A. Robison, R. W. Butcher and E. W. Sutherland, in Cyclic AMP (Academic Press, New York, 1971) p 378.

(37) J. F. Kuo, T. P. Lee, R. L. Reyes, K. G. Walton, T. E. Donnelly, Jr. and P. Greengard, J. Biol. Chem. 247 (1972) 16.

(38) J. W. Hadden, E. M. Hadden, M. K. Haddox and N. D. Goldberg, Proc. Nat. Acad. Sci. U.S. 69 (1972) 3024.

(39) J. Otten, G. S. Johnson and I. Pastan,
      Biochem. Biophys. Res. Commun. 44 (1971)
      1192.

(40) J. R. Sheppard, Nature (New Biol.) 236
      (1972) 14.

(41) J. Otten, J. Bader, G. S. Johnson and I.
      Pastan, J. Biol. Chem. 247 (1972) 1632.

(42) M. M. Burger, B. M. Bombik, B. M. Brecken-
      ridge and J. R. Sheppard, Nature (New Biol.)
      239 (1972) 161.

(43) C. E. Zeilig, R. A. Johnson, D. L. Friedman
      and E. W. Sutherland, J. Cell Biol. 55
      (1972) 296a.

(44) J. Otten, G. S. Johnson and I. Pastan, J.
      Biol. Chem. 247 (1972) 7082.

(45) J. J. Voorhees, E. A. Duell, L. J. Bass and
      E. R. Harrell, in: Journal of the National
      Cancer Institute Monograph Series, ed. B.
      K. Forscher and J. C. Houck, 1973, in press.

(46) E. J. Van Scott and E. M. Farber, in: Der-
      matology in General Medicine, ed. T. B.
      Fitzpatrick, K. A. Arndt, W. H. Clark, Jr.,
      A. Z. Eisen, E. J. Van Scott and J. H.
      Vaughan (McGraw Hill, 1971), p 219.

(47) J. J. Voorhees and E. A. Duell, in: Pso-
      riasis. Proceedings of the International
      Symposium, ed: E. M. Farber and A. J. Cox
      (Stanford University Press, Stanford, Calif.
      1971) p 305.

(48) J. W. Kebabian, J. Kuo and P. Greengard, in:
      Advances in Cyclic Nucleotide Research, Vol.
      2, ed. P. Greengard and G. A. Robison (Ra-
      ven Press, N.Y. 1972) p 131.

(49) S. L. Hsia, R. Wright, S. H. Mandy and
      K. M. Halprin, J. Invest. Dermatol. 59
      (1972) 109.

(50) G. R. Siggins, E. F. Battenberg, B. J. Hof-
      fer, F. E. Bloom and A. L. Steiner, Science
      179 (1973) 585.

(51) J. F. Whitfield, J. P. MacManus, D. J.
      Franks, D. J. Gillan and T. Youdale, Poc.
      Soc. Exp. Biol. Med. 137 (1971) 453.

(52) W. J. George, J. B. Palson, A. G. O'Toole
      and N. D. Goldberg, Poc. Nat. Acad. Sci.
      U.S. 66 (1970) 398.

(53) N. D. Goldberg, R. F. O'Dea and M. K. Had-
      dox, in: Advances in Cyclic Nucleotide
      Research, Vol. 3, ed. P. Greengard and
      G. A. Robison (Raven Press, N.Y. 1973) in
      press.

(54) M. Rodbell, L. Birnbaumer, S. L. Pohl and
      H. M. J. Krans, J. Biol. Chem. 246 (1971)
      1877.

(55) N. D. Goldberg, M. K. Haddox, D. K. Hartle
      and J. W. Hadden, in: Proceedings of the
      Fifth International Congress on Pharmacol-
      ogy, 1972, (Karger, Basel) in press.

(56) N. D. Goldberg, M. K. Haddox, R. Estensen,
      C. Lopez and J. W. Hadden, in: Cyclic AMP
      in Immune Response and Tumor Growth, eds.
      L. Lichtenstein, C. Parker, and W. Braun
      (Springer Verlag, New York, 1973) in press.

(57) L. Szodoray and I. Einleitung, Archiv fur
      klinische u. experimentelle Dermatologie,
      201 (1955) 581.

(58) A. E. Needham, in: Regeneration and Wound-
      Healing, ed. M. Abercrombie (Methuen & Co.
      Ltd. London, 1952) p 67.

(59) V. A. Ziboh and S. L. Hsia, J. Lipid Res. 13 (1972) 458.

(60) A. Rebora and G. Moretti, Arch. Derm. Forsch. 242 (1972) 323.

(61) G. S. Johnson and I. Pastan, J. National Cancer Inst. 48 (1972) 1377.

(62) J. R. Sheppard, Proc. Nat. Acad. Sci. U.S. 68 (1971) 1316.

(63) T. T. Puck, C. A. Waldren and A. W. Hsie, Proc. Nat. Acad. Sci. U.S. 69 (1972) 1943.

(64) A. W. Hsie and T. T. Puck, Proc. Nat. Acad. Sci. U.S. 68 (1971) 358.

(65) G. S. Johnson and I. Pastan, J. National Cancer Inst. 47 (1971) 1357.

(66) K. N. Prasad and A. Vernadakis, Exp. Cell Res. 70 (1972) 27.

(67) K. N. Prasad and B. Mandal, Exp. Cell Res. 74 (1972) 532.

(68) K. N. Prasad, J. C. Waymire and N. Weiner, Exp. Cell Res. 74 (1972) 110.

(69) J. C. Waymire, N. Weiner and K. N. Prasad, Proc. Nat. Acad. Sci. U.S. 69 (1972) 2241.

(70) K. N. Prasad, Nature (New Biol.) 236 (1972) 49.

(71) K. N. Prasad and J. R. Sheppard, Exp. Cell Res. 73 (1972) 436.

(72) P. Furmanski, D. J. Silverman and M. Lubin, Nature 233 (1971) 413.

(73) G. S. Johnson and I. Pastan, Nature (New Biol.) 237 (1972) 267.

(74) G. S. Johnson, R. M. Friedman and I. Pastan,
      Proc. Nat. Acad. Sci. U.S. 68 (1971) 425.

(75) M. Scheid, E. A. Boyse, E. A. Carswell and
      L. J. Old, J. Exp. Medicine 135 (1972) 938.

(76) J. R. Sheppard, in: Membranes and Viruses
      in Immunopathology (Academic Press, New
      York, 1972) p. 249.

(77) R. W. Holley, Proc. Nat. Acad. Sci. U.S.
      69 (1972) 2840.

(78) A. Hershko, P. Mamont, R. Shields and G. M.
      Tomkins, Nature (New Biol.) 232 (1971) 206.

(79) P. Mamont, A. Hershko, R. Kram, L. Schacter,
      J. Lust and G. M. Tomkins, Biochem. Biophys.
      Res. Commun. 48 (1972) 1378.

(80) G. M. Tomkins and T. D. Gelehrter, in: Bio-
      chemical Actions of Hormones, Ed. G. Lit-
      wack (Academic Press, New York, 1972) p 1.

(81) G. A. Robison, in: Medical Aspects of
      Prostaglandins and Cyclic AMP, Ed. R. Kahn
      (Academic Press, New York 1973) in press.

(82) V. R. Potter, in: Challenging Biological
      Problems, Ed. J. A. Behnke (Oxford Univer-
      sity Press, N.Y. 1972) p 52.

DISCUSSION

S.L. Hsia, University of Miami: Dr. Voorhees, naturally
I'd like to ask you a question about the disagreement in
your results and ours, on the adenyl cyclase activity
in the psoriatic skin and uninvolved skin. The specimen
that you examined included all the basal cells in the psoriatic
plaque. In other words, you have used a thicker specimen
that we have, and therefore you have included more dermis
in your specimen than the specimen we have looked at.
As you already indicated, there is an isoproterenol-sensitive
adenyl cyclase in the fibroblasts in the dermis, so, could
it be possible that the result you saw actually was in
part due to the activity of the dermis, therefore the response
in the dermis has covered up your lack of response in
the epidermis?

J.J. Voorhees, University of Michigan: Precisely.
That possibility is almost as equally as possible as the
possibility that you are assaying an enzyme that is in
much more dead cells in the involved than in the uninvolved
skin.

R.A. Hickie, University of Saskatchewan: I was wondering if anybody or if you have studied the effects of histamine
or kinins on cyclic AMP formation or adenyl cyclase, since
it's obviously local inflammatory response that you've seen
here. I think you alluded briefly to the effect of histamine
on mitosis.

J.J. Voorhees: We've never looked at kinins. We've
thought about it a great deal. The literature on brady-
kinin and what it does to cyclic AMP generation is rather
muddy, so we've stayed away from that. I belive that Dr.

Duell looked at histamine in broken cell preparations from mammalian epidermis early on and she did not find any effect of histamine on the epidermal adenyl cyclase. Now people have found effects in other tissues, but I understand that a lot of that data isn't reliable. Why, I don't know.

R.A. Hickie: In relation to this, it might be interesting to consider the possibility that histamine may change the permeability of the epidermal cells and somewhat allow cyclic AMP to get out and in this way dilate the blood vessels. As you mentioned, this was a characteristic action of cyclic AMP.

J.J. Voorhees: Yes, it sure might be. I don't know what histamine has got to do with psoriasis. That was an experimental tool, and I really wouldn't want to make any statements about histamine being involved in the pathophysiology of psoriasis. It's certainly an interesting possibility.

S. Belman, New York University: What effect does papaverine have on cyclic GMP levels?

J.J. Voorhees: Now that's an interesting question, because this gets us into Dr. Goldberg's area because in his measurements, as I understand it both papaverine and theophylline elevate both cyclic AMP and cyclic GMP, and it turns out out that in virtually every situation where he's looked at it, you usually see the cyclic AMP effect rather than the cyclic GMP effect, in other words, cyclic A dominates over cyclic G.

A. Wollenberger, Academy of Science of the G.D.R.: I have a question concerning your technique of taking samples of the epidermis. I don't know how you think about the anatomy of the skin but is it conceivable, that if you cut these pieces off that you might injure and thereby stimulate nerve fibers with subsequent release of transmitter and formation of second messenger, and that might perhaps falsify your results. Wouldn't it be perhaps possible

369

to freeze these pieces <u>in</u> <u>situ</u>?

J.J. Voorhees: Right. We could be injuring fibers
and stimulate transmitter release. That's a possibility.
We haven't ruled it out in or out. The clinical correlation
here actually sort of helps to rule that out. Wouldn't
you agree that if the disease situation seems to improve
in reponse to papaverine, that it was probably that way
in the patient. The other answer is that yes, we've thought
about freezing the tissue <u>in</u> <u>situ</u> because that's the way
a lot of pharmacologists do, but the problem you have
is in controlling the depth of the freezing and in order to
get the freezing controlled properly, I think that you
would wind up with a lot of scarring and ulceration.
The beauty of this technique is mainly because of the lack
of complications. We frequently make mistakes and go
too deep or too shallow or some such thing, but the data
shown today has been generated from about 310 patients,
and we have had an incidence of scarring of something
like about 1 or 2%. It's so low that we've actually written
people letters and asked them if they would care to do it
again, and most people would not mind it. Therefore,
this particular technique we happen to like, although it
is difficult to do.

S. Greer, University of Miami: I'd just like to comment
about your last slide. When lambda, the temperate bacterio-
phage of <u>Eschericia</u> <u>coli</u> enters a cell, it asks a similar
question, "Should I undergo the lytic (vegetative) cycle
or should I become a prophage to establish a lysogen-replicat-
ing in synchrony with the host cell"? This 'decision
has been found to depend on cAMP levels in the cell. One
should think about the states of integration of plasmids
(including viral-like particles) in cells as determining
the properties of cells, their life-style, their fate.

J.J. Voorhees: Right. We have even had a seminar
with the Microbiology Department on this tissue, thinking
about the possibility that sometimes viral diseases can mimic

polygenic inheritance. I can't make any statements about that. I know of an individual somewhere in lower Indiana who as far as I know has never published a paper, but claims to have seen C-type particles in psoriatic tissue. Now, I haven't made a rigorous investigation of psoriatic tissue because we use our electron microscope just as a quality control tool, but there could be viral particles in psoriatic tissue. On the other hand it could be viral disease without visible particles, I mean, really, this hasn't been looked at, if that's what you're getting at. But I think it's a nice suggestion.

R. Leif, Papanicolaou Cancer Research Institute:
Just a final comment. I think some of this problem of contamination with dermis could be solved by using cell dissociation and cell separation techniques. It is quite possible that in some of the previous papers where there have been conflicting results, these may be the result of different cells having different quantities of cyclic AMP, and that tissue culture cells are probably heterogenous. I think that it would be advisable to simplify the subject by performing these studies on pure cells in the same stage of the cell cycle.

J.J. Voorhees: Right, one does this, for example by using preparative cell electropheresis as has recently been shown to be capable of separating B and T lymphocytes. That would be fine. Now, if you dissociate the cells, I would guess that you would disrupt the cell surface and that might be a problem. Yes, it's a good idea, but you've got to remember that in the process of all of this that the cyclic AMP is going down, and the cyclic GMP might be going up, plus one must consider the number of cells that you're going to obtain for adenylate cyclase assay. This type of work is not easy. I think that's it's a great idea but I wouldn't care to try it.

S.L. Hsia: For this particular purpose, I would love to do some tissue culture work, to do some other studies

to differentiate between these cells and a normal cell.
Using this type medium, I think there are many pitfalls.
As you well realize, when you culture cells, they do
not retain all the characteristics of where you got them from.

J.J. Voorhees: Well, to do the best of my knowledge
nobody has ever cultured a human adult epidermal cell
for more than a few days and the number of cells one gets
is very small, impossible for biochemistry.

S. Belman: In the abstract you mentioned some work
with phorbol ester. Can you give us the data on that?

J.J. Voorhees: Right. The data on the phorbol ester
is fundamentally this. There is a diurnal variation in cyclic
AMP levels in the epidermis, as shown by F. Marks and
in Heidelberg, and we have done two rather large experiments
on this issue. In the first experiment, we found a rather
marked inhibition of the $G_1 \rightarrow S$ flow after the injection when
the experiments were done around the clock. We did
it a second time using even more animals, but the experimental
set-up was such that we worked during more of the daylight
hours only until midnight or so, so we were out of phase
with the first experiment and there the data was less convinc-
ing. In other words, we had a depression in the $G_1 \rightarrow S$
flow after IPR, but the depression was not statistically significant in the second experiment. So there's an indication
that IPR stimulated cyclic AMP accumation slows the $G_1 \rightarrow S$
flow, but the data is not hard at this moment.

H. Montes de Oca, University of Miami: I would
like to comment on your statement that epithelial cells cannot
be cultured. At present I have several cultures of human
skin from different donors which, at the third split, still
maintain typical epithelial morphology. Under proper culture
conditions, these cultures produce melanin and keratin.

J.J. Voorhees: Right. Well, that's fine. We are growing
epithelial cells as well, and are in the process of developing

enzymatic profiles to be able to distinguish epithelial
cells from fibroblasts, because after they've been around
awhile they look sort of the same. We feel that we're going
to be rather close to being able to do this very shortly,
but right at the moment there isn't anyone that I know of,
in the case of the surface line epithelium type work who
has really done this rigorously enough to use that as an
experimental cell culture system. Now you may have already
done this, I don't know.